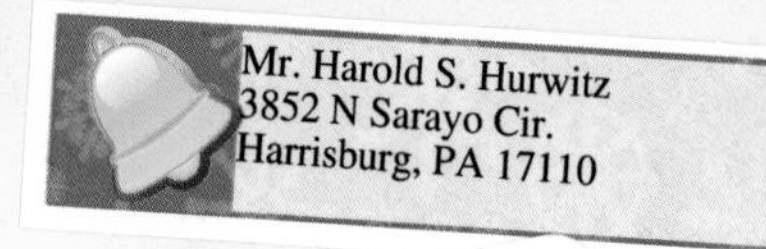
Mr. Harold S. Hurwitz
3852 N Sarayo Cir.
Harrisburg, PA 17110

D1074175

HOW TO GET A GOOD NIGHT'S SLEEP

By the same author:

YOU LIVE AS YOU BREATHE
COMMON SENSE CORONARY CARE AND PREVENTION
YOUR LIFE TO ENJOY
MR. EXECUTIVE: KEEP WELL—LIVE LONGER
YOU CAN INCREASE YOUR HEART POWER
LIVE LONGER AND ENJOY IT
THE DOCTOR LOOKS AT LIFE
HOW TO STOP KILLING YOURSELF
HEART WORRY AND ITS CURE
WHAT YOU CAN DO FOR ANGINA PECTORIS AND CORONARY OCCLUSION
WHAT YOU CAN DO FOR HIGH BLOOD PRESSURE
HOW TO MASTER YOUR FEARS
HOW TO KEEP FIT WITHOUT EXERCISE
HOW TO ADD YEARS TO YOUR LIFE
HEART DISEASE IS CURABLE
MORE YEARS FOR THE ASKING

HOW TO GET A GOOD NIGHT'S SLEEP

peter j. steincrohn, m.d.

HENRY REGNERY COMPANY · Chicago

LIBRARY OF CONGRESS CATALOG CARD NUMBER: 68-18275
MANUFACTURED IN THE UNITED STATES OF AMERICA

Dedicated

to

Tossers, snorers, groaners,
Pillow-punchers, sleep-talkers, clock-watchers,
Twisters-and-turners, counters-of-sheep;

to

Worry-ridden, tension-filled insomniacs
Lying there wide-eyed night after night;

to

100,000,000 Americans
Who have said, are saying or will say:
"How'll I ever get through tomorrow?"

Contents

Introduction 1

I | SLEEPMANSHIP IN HEALTH

1 | Common Beliefs and Misbeliefs About Sleep 9

2 | ABC's of Sleep Physiology 20

3 | Sleep Needs for Children,
Adolescents, Adults, the Elderly 28

4 | Narcolepsy: Enemy of Insomnia 39

5 | Leg Jitters: Insomnia's First Lieutenant 48

6 | Dreams, Nightmares, Sleepwalking, Snoring 57

7 | Some Common Causes of Insomnia 72

8 | Serendipity and Sleep 85

II | SLEEPMANSHIP IN ILLNESS

9 | Sleep and Heart Disease 91

10 | Sleep and Chronic Anxiety 105

11 | Sleep and Ulcer Trouble 119

12 | Sleep and Thyroid Disorders 125

13 | Sleep and Allergies ... 131

14 | Sleep and the Menopause ... 137

15 | Sleep and Mental Disorders ... 139

III | SLEEPMANSHIP: FACTS, FICTION, FANCIES

16 | Sleep: Assorted Facts and Fiction ... 151

17 | Bedside Advice from Readers ... 170

IV | SLEEPMANSHIP: PRACTICAL METHODS

18 | The Basic Strategy for Overcoming Insomnia ... 183

19 | Practical Pointers for Overcoming Insomnia ... 192

20 | Closing Note: The Outlook ... 207

"In its many forms, insomnia probably constitutes one of mankind's most subtle tortures . . ."

—U.S. Department of Health and Welfare

"Nothing in all the range of human complaints excites my sympathy so much as sleeplessness."

—Arthur E. Hertzler, M.D.

"Modern cure for insomnia: counting sheep with a Univac."

—Peter J. Steincrohn

Introduction

HAVE YOU SURRENDERED TO INSOMNIA? Do you now accept loss of sleep, with its consequent fatigue, loss of energy, deadened reflexes, lack of zest, increased irritability and decreased ambition, as one of the inevitable consequences of modern existence?

Do you say, "I didn't sleep a wink last night," and act like a martyr who has had all the fight taken out of him? Or do you rebel? Are you willing to fight on for a good night's sleep?

If you are still game, please believe me when I say there is much you can do to overcome your sleep problems. I reiterate this in spite of all you hear from scientists who keep saying, "There's so much we still don't know about sleep."

Too many have become convinced that sleep is an overrated commodity, that it is not as necessary as most people think. Arnold Bennett was only one of many who preached this doctrine. Napoleon said that the eight-hour sleep was for idiots. Many modern experimenters and researchers lull us into acceptance of insomnia by saying that there is no overall sleep formula.

Perhaps you, like many other Americans, consider it to be a waste of life itself to stay in bed longer than "necessary." You have come to begrudge the hours spent there; you count them as a loss. It hurts your conscience to throw hours onto the heap of unconscious existence.

For this reason growing youths often get night after

night only the bare essentials of mind-repair produced by sleep; housewives who stay up into the early hours for the late-late or early-early TV shows virtually drag themselves out of bed in time to make breakfast for their husbands and send the kids off to school; and businessmen who trudge home very late from lodge meetings, poker games or plain parties get up groggy-eyed to a busy day without the necessary hours of energy-renewal the human body requires.

Much of today's unrecognized inefficiency is due to lack of sleep, to fatigue. Pray that the man whose car approaches you at seventy miles per hour on the highway has had a good night's sleep. Otherwise, your life is hostage to his drowsiness.

Chronic fatigue is a by-product of sleeplessness, and it is therefore a common symptom of insomnia. No day goes by in which the doctor doesn't hear this complaint from some patients. And unless he delves carefully into his patient's history and discovers chronic sleep-lack, he may falsely pin guilt on the innocent, saying that the fatigue is due to tension in the office or home, anemia, poor diet, anxiety or to actual organic illness.

Therefore, I suggest that you forget Napoleon and the more modern, well-meaning, red-blooded heroes who skip about bragging that they get along on very little sleep. Look only to yourself. Take inventory of your personal sleeping habits and of your own reactions to lack of sufficient sleep.

How do you feel? Tired? (And you don't know why?) Irritable? (And you can't put your finger on the reason?) Unambitious? (Yet you wanted so much to take on the new project?) Sleepy in the afternoon? You wonder how you will get through the day? (Yet you haven't even considered lack of sufficient sleep as a cause?)

Like food and water, sleep is one of the elements essential for survival. Chronic loss of sleep can be as devastating to body and spirit as chronic starvation or water deprivation. In fact, lack of sleep can make your life a succession of "daymares." Perhaps they're not so acutely frightening as nightmares; nevertheless, they have a deadening impact. Unfrightening, they are devitalizing. Sleep is essential for survival itself.

Far from being a luxury, sleep is a prime necessity for efficient and enjoyable existence. Sleep is not a loss-in-living. It is an important cog in the chain that binds day to day and night to night.

Whether one tries to discover it on the Indian fakir's bed of nails or on Western man's bed of down-feathers, the trigger-mechanism that produces this steadily recurring brain-numbing still eludes us. Sleep remains a stubborn enigma. All we know is that we need it.

Much has been postulated and studied and postulated again, but sleep remains the ever recurring daily mystery. So far every clue has been only a tantalizing promise. Scientific investigation has steadily hacked out a beginning path. But the thick underbrush of countless theories, superstitions and old wives' tales obscures our vision and interrupts our progress toward eventual solution.

Of course, we must persevere. The future will bring us our answer. But when is the future? The twenty-fifth century? Next year? Next month? The day after tomorrow? The future is a vague promise. And if you are interested in sleep, the day after tomorrow is too far away. You want to be fully equipped to meet its challenge tonight, not tomorrow night.

In this book I propose to show what sleep is and why it is so important to you. Consider this book a practical stopgap, a specific antidote against the poison of insomnia until electronics (or some other invention) comes along to make sleep as old-fashioned as the caveman's prolonged snoozing in an age when there was little to do but sleep.

You will learn about the various sleep theories; about that strange, rude bedfellow called insomnia; about naps; about tranquilizers and sleeping pills.

I will tell you about narcolepsy, the reverse of insomnia, the sufferers of which have to fight to stay awake.

Do you suffer from the Restless Leg syndrome? Do you snore, sleepwalk or have nightmares? Are you concerned about your dreams?

Do you sleep with your wife (or your husband) and wish you had the nerve to say, "Darling, don't you think we ought to have twin beds?" (You will learn that togetherness can be overdone.)

Are you concerned (or, worse still, unconcerned) about your sleeping equipment? Beds, mattresses, pillows, blankets, bedroom location and a score of other collaterals are the forgotten materiél of comfortable daily existence.

I will discuss sleep-needs during illness brought on by heart ailments, ulcers, hyperthyroidism, anxiety states, allergies, mental disorders, menopause, hiatal hernia, hyperventilation, prostate disease and Parkinson's and other diseases.

Above all, I will tell you how to get a good night's sleep. *How to Get a Good Night's Sleep* is a "how to" rather than a "what's what" book. Undoubtedly you are more interested in ways to overcome stubborn insomnia than in reading a speculative dissertation on various sleep theories. You will find no pretensions here about cause and effect. Nobody has yet solved the basic mystery of what causes sleep or even of what it is.

But observations over many years in the practice of medicine have revealed to me several practical methods for overcoming, or at least neutralizing, insomnia. In this book, therefore, I will try to show you "how to."

If you are one of the millions who yearn for nightly surcease from daily cares, you should concentrate on the problem that interests us here and now: insomnia. You should then do something about it. Don't just lie there, night after night, waiting endlessly for some genie to bring gentle sleep to your troubled mind.

Remember General Anthony C. McAuliffe's answer to the German request that he surrender at Bastogne:

"Nuts," he said.

Let us adopt that as our rallying cry in the fight against insomnia. Rather than knuckle under we should knuckle up to it. If we can say "nuts" to insomnia—and mean it—the battle is ours.

Sleepmanship in Health | I

1 | Common Beliefs and Misbeliefs About Sleep

IF YOU NEED A GOOD NIGHT'S SLEEP, it is unlikely that you are especially interested in whether your sleep loss is due to dysfunction of a sleep center in the brain, to chemical imbalance in the blood, to a "cut-off" in nerve-muscle interactions or to any of several other still unproved theories.

Your basic desire is to learn how to get enough sleep to prepare you for the coming day. According to many polls, the sleep problem called insomnia bedevils, has bedeviled or will bedevil at least one out of two Americans—man and boy, woman and girl, that adds up to at least 100,000,000 of us. On many a night, instead of being cozily cuddled in the arms of Morpheus, you have twisted and turned to free yourself from the bonds of insomnia.

Are you getting sufficient sleep? The answer may not be as apparent as you believe. I have known many chronically tired and exhausted patients who blamed their sub-par existence on overwork, lack of vitamins, worry and scores of other causes when insomnia was really the culprit.

Many of these people suffered from chronic fatigue and listlessness because they were getting only six hours of sleep a night when they actually required eight or nine. Somewhere they had read or heard that most of us sleep our lives away, so they forced themselves to stay awake late night after night. To stiffen this self-imposed sentence of wakefulness, insomnia crept in to drain their vital energy.

Either they watched the late-late-late shows on TV or they read until 2 A.M.; in either case, they dragged themselves out of bed at 7 A.M. The simple prescription of two added hours of sleep was all they needed to feel full of vigor and life.

Although it is true that some people require little sleep, they are the fortunate minority. I know a healthy man in his mid-sixties who swears that he has not averaged more than five hours of sleep a night since adulthood, yet he is surfeited with energy.

For most of us, however, this regime would change potentially efficient beings into unfeeling zombies wandering through their daily tasks like automatons.

If experience has convinced you that you do not thrive on the five to six hour nightly routine of sleep, you had better keep to your schedule of eight to nine hours to ensure twelve months of feeling rested, fit and alive during your waking hours. This makes more sense than being bogged down by loss of interest, chronic fatigue and a daily battle to keep your eyelids pried apart.

By experiment find your own particular requirement. If you have been sleeping five to six hours nightly, try adding an hour or two each day for a week. Does the additional rest contribute to your well-being? Then wisdom dictates that you adopt this new schedule permanently.

On the other hand, perhaps you really have been wasting valuable time. Perhaps you have been sleeping too much. Try cutting down to seven hours nightly, then to six. If you do well on this new regime, you will have captured more hours in which to do all the things you want to do.

All this time I have been presuming that you have little

trouble in sleeping. You just plop into bed and off you go into the sublime state of blissful slumber, sweet dreams and temporary oblivion.

For many insomniacs this would be heaven itself.

A REAL PROBLEM

Make no excuses for being too sleep-conscious.

Greater men and women than you and I have had a life-long tussle with insomnia. However ridiculous your attempts to court sleep may seem, you may be sure that somewhere, sometime a frustrated human being is being more ludicrous and absurd.

Insomnia is not an inconsiderable speck of a problem. I wish I could dismiss it as easily as did Mark Twain, who said, "If you can't sleep, try lying on the end of the bed—then you might drop off."

But neither can I accept the other extreme: too much absorption in the need for a good night's sleep. For example, Louis XIV of France owned 413 beds, and Ben Franklin had four in his bedroom and rotated upon them as each became warm.

How much sleep you or I require is an intensely personal problem that only you or I can solve. In spite of what Napoleon (some say Aristotle) said—"Six hours of sleep for a man, seven for a woman and eight for a fool"—do not be fooled. If Pope Leo XIII, who required only three hours of sleep nightly, would have felt he was wasting time lolling in bed for six hours, Woodrow Wilson, exhausted unless he had nine hours' sleep, would not have agreed that even eight hours was sufficient.

MAYBE YOU NEED MORE SLEEP

I do not agree with Napoleon, Aristotle or anyone who pronounces us fools if we require at least eight hours of sleep. I fall within the eight to nine hour range. For me, the most trying part of getting up early the next morning is thinking about it late the night before.

In fact, I go along with the wisdom of the saying, "For most people it is true that if they sleep for almost half of their lives, they will enjoy the other half twice as much."

After a week of nightly sleep debits, however much I try to philosophize, I become irritable, dull and listless. I cannot go along with Arnold Bennett's theory that five to six hours are sufficient, even if he tempts you with simple arithmetic: if you sleep only six hours nightly, you gain 750–800 hours —the equivalent of an extra month of living—per year. Quite a bonus!

But suppose that extra month is spent while befogged, bedraggled and befuddled? Where is the gain? How can those of us who need more sleep cut corners? How can we heavy-lids compare ourselves to the light-lids who make jokes about insomnia?

For example, Stephen Leacock tells a story to prove that "this insomnia business is about 90 per cent nonsense." When he was a young man living in a boarding house in Toronto, his brother George came to visit him. Since there was no spare room, they had to share one bed. In the morning both complained that they had not slept a wink. "Then we put our heads up from the bedclothes and saw that the bed was covered with plaster. The ceiling had fallen on us in the night. But we hadn't noticed it. We had 'insomnia.' "

Not only do we heavy-lids suffer tortures indescribable when we haven't had our full sleep-quota night after night, we are often the targets of barbs thrown by those who suspect that there is a neurotic basis for our urge to sleep well. They say that we are unable to circumvent or meet our daily problems so we try to find solace in prolonged sleep, that because of our tensions we must recuperate in a warm, relaxed, uterine state, freed of our waking responsibilities.

Theories and explanations of the mystery of sleep continue to be put forth with resourcefulness and imagination. But wakefulness and sleep remain as basic and inevitable as the extremes of heat and cold, sunset and sunrise, tide in and tide out, black and white, love and hate. Speculate all we will on thermal units, skies, water, colors, human emotions and sleep: enigmas they still remain.

THERE ARE MANY THEORIES

Scientists continue to study the nature and cause of sleep and wakefulness. Some day we shall have the true answers. How sleep originates. Where it originates. Why it is essential.

One of the oldest theories I can recall is the neuron theory. In this, the synapses, or points of contact of the nerves, and the nerve cells in the brain lose contact through a process of retraction. It is as if while shaking hands with a person, you withdrew your extended fingers. Or it's as if some sort of electrical circuit was broken. The loss of contact between nerve ends and brain is supposed to produce sleep. But however interesting it is as a theory, it hasn't yet been proved.

Some prefer the cerebral ischemic theory. Briefly, the

theory is that owing to fatigue of the vasomotor center in the brain that regulates the dilation and contraction of blood vessels, there is widespread dilation of the blood vessels of the skin. The dilation reduces blood flow in the brain itself and is primarily responsible for the onset of sleep. Yet other scientists say in refutation that there is no diminution of blood flow during sleep. The theory remains controversial and unproved.

A chemical theory intrigued the medical profession for a long while: excess lactic acid formed when one became tired was supposed to suppress the brain's activities and produce sleep. However, brilliant investigators in the opposition camp disagree. They say you don't have to be tired to sleep, and that you may be completely exhausted and still be unable to sleep.

An even more recent chemical theory says that a substance called "hypnotoxin" is the actual cause of sleep. The tired brain itself is supposed to manufacture it. We are awaiting more proof before we accept this theory.

The Russian scientist Pavlov had a theory, too: that certain stimuli—boredom, a dull lecture, a quiet, even voice—cause the entire cortex of the brain to slow down. But he did not believe that the entire brain goes to sleep. It is for this reason that a mother can sleep undisturbed through a thunderstorm yet hear the tiny cry of her baby.

MORE THEORIES

Still another theory is that a center in the brain-stem called the diencephalon is the source of sleep. It has been found that when a tumor grows in this region, or when its center is mildly stimulated with electrical current or by a drug, sleep follows. According to many students of the sleep problem, there is evidence that this theory is a strong one.

Dr. Nathaniel Kleitman, University of Chicago physiologist and recognized authority on the study of sleep, has advanced the theory that sleep is the result of a reduction in the impulses that come from the muscles of the body to the brain, causing an inactivity of the brain's cells. He believes that the fatigue of the mechanism that mediates the tone between muscle and nerve, with consequent suppression of the impulses from the muscle, is the most important factor in producing sleep. He thinks that loss of muscle tone is invariably a prelude to sleep. For example, if you lie down when you're very sleepy, you will fall asleep; but if you walk when you are sleepy, you will stay awake. It is as simple as that—or we hope it is.

There are other theories. Studies on monkeys were said to show that there is a "waking center" in the back part of the hypothalamus section of the brain. An investigator who experimented on rats discovered what he considers to be a "sleep center" in the hypothalamus, and he believes that this sleeping center in some way inhibits the activity of the waking center, thus bringing on sleep.

When one considers how bored and sleepy one gets after immersing oneself in these variegated theories, it seems that there may well be some truth in Pavlov's sleep theory!

SLEEP STILL AN ENIGMA

Because of the confusion of theories about sleep and its stubborn resistance to the scientific probings of man in his laboratory, I see and listen, with open eyes and ears, to the unscientific experiments and beliefs of the guinea pigs themselves: to the men, women and children who have had bouts with insomnia and think they have discovered a winning formula. (In Chapter 17 I will record many of their suggestions.)

I believe I could cure millions of insomniacs without writing another line of this book if I could get them to believe and put it into practice what Emerson said: "Those only can sleep who do not care to sleep well."

But you know and I know that this simple cure is difficult to attain. How can you convince a sleepless man at 2 A.M. to forget about the "big day" he has tomorrow? The harder he tries to sleep, the tighter he shuts his eyes, the more elusive becomes the restful slumber he craves. It is not at all easy to affect nonchalance when you are anchored in the mire of fatigue and frustration caused by sleep loss.

VARYING REACTIONS TO INSOMNIA

People are bound to go to extremes when they are convinced they have the solution to any stubborn problem. Consider the poet Amy Lowell. She insisted that she needed absolute quiet in order to sleep well. When she stayed at a hotel, she is said to have hired five rooms for the night: one to sleep in and an empty one on each side, above and below. That is what I call wrapping oneself in a cocoon—an expensive one, at that.

Charles Dickens carried a compass with him when he was away from home so that he could move his bed to allow his head to point north. He said he slept with his head north because of the theory that magnetic currents ran north and south between the poles. He reasoned, therefore, that by allowing these currents to flow through the body in a straight line he could overcome insomnia. Silly? Until actually disproved beyond a doubt, it isn't any more preposterous than scientific, unproved observations on sleep.

Dr. E.B. Foote, in *Plain Home Talk* (published in 1870), had some interesting observations on magnetic influences:

> I have looked in vain in the writings of medical men and physiologists for any rational reason why man should lie down at night and rise with the sun. . . . Most persons are ready to attribute any other cause than the true one.
>
> Therefore, there is great need of new light on this subject—something which will appeal to the *reason* of men, and demonstrate the fact that one hour of sleep at night is worth more than three after the sun has risen.
>
> From the investigations I have made, I have come to the conclusion that during the day the magnetic or electric currents from the sun predominate, and descending perpendicularly or obliquely the upright body is brought in harmony with the descending currents; while at night the magnetic or electric currents of the earth predominate, and flow from north to south horizontally, in consequence of which the human body should be in a recumbent position, with head to the north, in order to preserve the harmonious circulation of the nervo-electric fluids.
>
> . . . Then, there are a few whose strong nervous organizations appear to resist all such influences, but the continual dropping of water wears away a stone, and these exceptions finally favor the truth of this philosophy. The sun exerts a powerful magnetic influence on the earth, arousing all animal life to activity, from the merest insect to the noblest work of God.
>
> The fowls of the air, the beasts of the field and all human beings who obey the laws of nature, feel inspired

> with new life when the golden rays of the rising sun radiate from the east. The activity of animal fluids increases till he reaches his meridian, and then gradually decreases until he sinks to rest in the west.
>
> When "Old Sol" retires, the colder magnetic currents of the earth prevail with greater power; animal life becomes more sluggish; the wearied body seeks repose; and the most perfect repose is obtained by reclining in a position consonant with the earth's currents.

Aristotle said he was sorry he was not an insomniac. He believed that his time was wasted in sleep, and that lying awake wishing that one could sleep was a waste of time. He said that people are too afraid of insomnia and that it can be put to good use and be fun. Aristotle did not realize that his contempt for insomnia was what drove it from his bed and made him a good sleeper. His is the most reliable way to win at the game of Sleepmanship.

I recall when I was still in my teens reading about a great potentate, reputedly the richest man in the world, who promised he would give away half his riches to the first person who would offer him the cure for his insomnia. I went to bed that night determined to think of a formula that would help the great man and enrich me. Unfortunately, I fell right off to sleep. (Had I been an insomniac, I might have been the world's second richest man.)

In succeeding years I read no headlines announcing the cure. Probably the lucky fellow stumbled upon some simple cure that didn't cost him a dime: something like a cup of hot water before retiring or sleeping on a mattress instead of on a tiger rug spread out on the floor of his palace bedroom. Most likely of all, he learned "not to care" whether he slept or not.

INSOMNIA A PERSONAL PROBLEM

So many factors enter into the problem of insomnia—emotional, physical, psychological. Sometimes the doctor can help; often the patient himself must find the answer. Each one with intractable insomnia has a personal problem to overcome. There is no blanket-treatment that will cover everyone, make them comfortable and put them to sleep.

Nevertheless, there is an answer for many people, as you will find out later in this book.

2 | ABC's of Sleep Physiology

INSOMNIA IS MORE THAN an eight-letter word. It is made up, in various combinations, of all twenty-six letters of the alphabet from A (anxiety) to Z (zealousness). Every second American has at some time resented its indignities. Its causes and cures are numberless. It bedevils the rich and the poor, the healthy and the sick, the young and the old—male and female. It is the uninvited guest who insists on staying overnight—night after night.

Insomnia is a strange bedfellow. It mimics and it mocks. The following day it produces discomforts that range from an innocent yawn to soul-deadening irritability and inefficiency. It is more stubborn than yielding. It may be the forerunner of a severe mental breakdown or only the herald of the common complaint "I've got to catch up on my sleep."

One of the many excellent and terse definitions of insomnia is "prolonged failure to procure sufficient sleep necessary to maintain health and well-being."

Insomnia usually takes one of three forms: (1) inability to fall asleep on retiring; (2) frequent awakening (for minutes or hours) during the night; (3) getting up too early, before attaining sufficient sleep.

But you will cope with insomnia more successfully if you first know some basic facts about sleep itself.

Many physiological changes occur when you sleep. Your blood pressure declines ten to thirty points. It reaches its lowest level about the fourth hour, remaining at that level until just before you awaken, when it begins to rise again. When you have an exciting dream, your pressure may leap to 180–200. You can understand, therefore, why people who already have high blood pressure are in some danger if they are subject to dreams and nightmares that excite them. (More about this in Chapter 6.)

While you're asleep, your pulse rate is slowed ten to thirty beats; your basal metabolism is lowered about 15 per cent; even your temperature falls a bit. Your respirations are lowered and sometimes become irregular. Your muscle tone falls below normal, and reflexes such as the knee-jerk no longer operate. Your eyeballs turn upward and outward, and your urine volume lessens.

Your sweat glands overwork during sleep, sometimes secreting as much per hour as when you exercise strenuously. Your stomach may contract more vigorously, but your rate of digestion is about the same as when you are awake. The secretions of the glands that lubricate the eyes and throat are reduced.

The depth of your sleep varies from hour to hour. As a rule the sleep you get during the day is lighter than that obtained at night. Dreams occur in light sleep and not in deep sleep. The body is not completely at rest during sleep. You may turn as many as twenty-five or thirty times, and you cannot judge the quality of your sleep by the number of times you have turned. For example, if you say that you tossed all night, during eight hours in bed you may have "tossed" for a total of only three to five minutes. A normal person will spend about 20 per cent of the night in the dreaming stage; 60 per cent in intermediate stages; and 20 per cent in deep, non-dreaming sleep.

HOW CAN WE BE SURE YOU ARE ASLEEP?

How can we tell that a person is really asleep? He might be able to fool us if we merely observe him apparently fast asleep in bed, but not if we attach some electrodes to his head and take an electroencephalogram. These brain-wave tracings show specific changes during natural sleep (incidentally, such changes do not occur during hypnosis).

In sleep there is a disappearance of alpha waves (which may also disappear during concentration and excitement). When a person falls asleep his brain waves change from steady alpha waves to bursts of alpha waves, which then stop altogether. The alpha waves are followed by spindle waves, delta waves, rollers, fine fast ripples and, finally, by a disappearance of all important rhythms.

A study of brain waves indicates that sleep induced by sleeping drugs is not much different from natural sleep. It also indicates that each time you turn over in sleep your slumber becomes lighter just before you move and deeper when the movement is completed. If you have recently moved in sleep, you are more easily awakened by a noise than if you have been sleeping motionless.

Short dreams and deep sleep come early in the night. You are not totally unconscious when you are asleep. Your brain and sense organs remain alert to respond to signals of danger.

Many people wonder why they feel less refreshed if they wake in the morning and go to sleep again before they get up than if they open their eyes and get right out of bed. The reason is that when one wakes from regular sleep in the morning, it is from a light sleep, but when one then goes to sleep again, one wakes from a heavy sleep. When we are asleep, we are constantly changing from light sleep to deep sleep and back again. Very often we are almost awake when asleep.

Although all of your muscles are relaxed during sleep, there is some remaining tonicity in the eyelid and jaw muscles and, fortunately, in the sphincter muscles of the rectum and urinary bladder. Sensory perception is reduced.

Normal sleep is not one deep valley of black oblivion. However blanketed in seeming unconsciousness, the mind never stops functioning. As if on an elevator, the mind ascends and descends to varying levels of consciousness. The EEG or electroencephalograph is the brain-wave recording device that has lifted the curtain—though not yet completely—on many of the mysteries of sleep.

On the graphs, recorded with the help of electrodes attached to the human volunteer guinea pig's skull, we learn that during wakefulness brain waves are irregular, rapid and shallow. As relaxation and dimness of conscious thought set in, the new pattern of the alpha rhythm of lessened cycles per second occurs.

Then the alpha waves become smaller as the sleeper sinks into Stage 1, the first level of sleep. If you wake him now, he will say he was not really asleep.

After the preliminary minutes in Stage 1, he takes the elevator down to the second level, Stage 2. His brain waves have changed. Now they come in quick bursts in the shape of the spindles I mentioned above. His sleep is deeper, but not yet deep. Nature again pushes the button, and the elevator descends another level to Stage 3. He is now relaxed, his heart slows, he breathes regularly and his temperature falls. The EEG waves now occur only about once every second.

At last (about a half-hour after he has fallen asleep) he sinks to Stage 4, the deepest sleep level. Sleep-wise he is now on the ground floor. The EEG exhibits large, lazy brain waves called delta waves. The sleeper is "dead asleep."

But even normal sleep is a restless sort of critter. In about half an hour he has drifted upward into the lighter sleep levels again. In another hour he may be close to waking, though he in fact doesn't. After some time in Stage 1 he will descend again to Stage 4. He takes this round trip on our metaphorical elevator at least four or five times nightly.

Although the delta stage is like deepest unconsciousness, the brain is not entirely inactive. Normal sleep approximates unconsciousness, but chiefly it resembles it. The brain of the sleeper is aware of various stimuli to which the brain of the unconscious person is oblivious. For example, during normal sleep one will awaken when discomfort or pain breaks through. Stirring or complete wakefulness may occur in answer to visual, auditory or olfactory signals: a light shining on the eyelids, a gunshot or roll of thunder, the smell of smoke. One stays awake or falls back to sleep depending on the intensity or importance of the waking stimulus.

As I said above, few persons remain completely motionless during sleep ("sleep like a log") because nature finds that changing position during sleep prevents pooling of blood in dependent organs and improves muscle tone. Turning also helps respiration by unsplinting compressed chest muscles, allowing for better exchange of oxygen and carbon dioxide in the smaller alveoli of the lungs.

Blood pressure is not always at its *lowest* level during deepest sleep, but sleep is usually associated with some fall in blood pressure. Deep sleep, however, produces the most *regular* blood pressure and respiration. Blood pressure may rise, fall or remain unchanged during dreams. The higher the waking pressure, the greater the fall during sleep.

One important discovery is that REM (rapid eye movement) is a signal of dreaming. If you are awakened just after a REM period, you will recall your dream vividly. If you wake at other times, your recollections will be vague, or absent.

In *Facts on Sleep* Dr. S.B. Whitehead gives a number of interesting details. The most prolific years for dreaming are between the ages of twenty and twenty-five. The average time taken to fall asleep is fourteen minutes. Fat people require less sleep than thin. We spend an average of 110 days in bed per year. Between the ages of twenty and sixty-five most of us spend approximately fifteen years asleep.

Each eight-hour sleep 527 muscles relax; we change position approximately 24 times and breathe about 6,525 times. Dr. Whitehead has even measured the average noise of a snore: fifty-eight decibels at four feet.

According to Dr. Kleitman, there are three predominant rhythms of sleep.

Type one is the "morning type." You jump out of bed, fully awake and raring to go. You are full of verve and plans for the day while the rest of the family are still wiping cobwebs of sleep out of their eyes. You slow up in late afternoon and come almost to a full stop in the evening. But the "morning sleepyheads" are now at their peak. They want to go and do things; you are ready for bed.

Type two is the "evening type." The alarm clock is your mortal enemy. You have to drag yourself out of bed and to the office. Comes the afternoon, and you are the sparkplug of the organization just when the others are beginning to wilt. And at night you are the one who hates to take leave of guests until long after midnight because you are in full mental and physical stride.

If you are type three, you are fortunate. When you fit into this classification, you are in full stride morning and night—and have only a moderate midday letdown to contend with.

Ask yourself this question: "How much sleep do I really need?" Finding the correct answer is worthwhile. Your health, efficiency and happiness depend on it.

If you have never tried getting along on less sleep, try it for a week. If you thrive on it, there is your "open sesame" to a longer life. But let us assume that you *need* those eight hours. What to do about it?

First, as mentioned earlier, find your rhythm. If you are an early-to-bed, early-to-rise individual or a late-to-bed, late-to-rise sort of person, recognize yourself for what you are.

If you are fortunate, you will be able to fit yourself to the job that least interferes with your sleep rhythm. If you are an early bird, schedule most of the important work for the first hours of the day—before afternoon and evening lassitude benumbs your brain and body.

If you are a late bird, don't schedule your productive labor until late morning or afternoon. There is nobody so inefficient as the early-morning grouch whose surliness is due to sleepiness and low vitality.

And what is perhaps most important: do not forget the energy-recharging value of naps. Whatever your sleep cycle, a Sunday afternoon nap acts as a weekly restorative. If you are the early riser who fades out in the evening, the after-luncheon or mid-afternoon nap acts as a shot of adrenaline to a person who needs stimulation to keep him going.

If you are the "death-of-the-party," try a pre-party nap sometime. Your friends won't recognize you around midnight. And you'll pinch yourself to make sure it's you.

The answer to the sleep problem seems to lie in the fact that there is no universal arithmetic applying to everyone. Each of us has to do his own adding and subtracting. But it is worth the trouble. Finding the right answer means much in living comfort and efficiency.

For some the physiology of sleep is as simple as ABC. But for millions of insomniacs the quest for the solution of the sleep problem stretches to the XYZ's. When you finish this book, I hope you will be closer to the first part of the alphabet than to the last.

3 | Sleep Needs for Children, Adolescents, Adults, the Elderly

ONE GALLUP POLL showed that 52 per cent of the people in the United States had occasional or frequent difficulty getting to sleep. People, of course, includes children, adolescents, adults and the elderly. The same poll found that the Old World (Holland, Britain, France, Sweden, Denmark, Norway) sleeps better than the New. For example, in Norway only 15 per cent of the population reports insomnia. But before there is a sudden exodus of sleepless Americans to Norway, let me warn that unless you leave behind your tensions, you will discover that your old bedfellow, insomnia, has accompanied you on your travels.

Only one out of four Scandinavians complained of insomnia and one out of three Frenchmen, yet every second American does.

Those who travel immediately sense that life in other countries goes on more slowly than in America. In England it may take you almost two hours to finish a pot of tea. During a stay in Italy I recall needing the services of a pharmacist to counteract the irritation caused by a speck of dust in my eye. Unfortunately, I needed help in the early afternoon. All the pharmacies I tried were locked up temporarily while the owners took their daily siesta.

But here in America you find people standing at a soda fountain gulping down a hamburger and a soft drink. It would be economic suicide for our "pharmacies" to close during lunch hour. Think of all the lunch sales (and the occasional eye-wash sale) they would lose.

And so it is with sleep. We sleep too fast, too. Unconsciously, we Americans seem to resent time lost in sleep. Perhaps that is one of the major causes for our sleeplessness as a nation.

On the other hand, perhaps we are more realistic than we realize. We do not run away from realities. Perhaps our realistic outlook is what makes one in two of us insomniacs at one time or another. After all, many people sleep overtime to escape reality.

Napoleon, who usually slept no longer than four hours, slept much longer after his defeats at Aspern and Waterloo. It has been said that a gambler can go many days and nights without sleep if he is winning. After a heavy losing streak, however, he can sleep for many days and nights at a time, just getting up to eat and take care of other physiological needs.

WHY WE NEED MORE SLEEP

There is an evolutional explanation of the need for less sleep that may explain the go-get-'em American's insomnia. The supporters of this sleep-wakefulness theory maintain that our primitive forebears slept practically the entire day around, getting up only to eat, procreate and perform other such basic functions. Life was dull, and there was no need to stay awake and become an integral part of the boredom of existence.

But during the slow evolution of man, as his higher brain centers became dominant, he invented interests and pleasures. He wanted to stay awake to enjoy them. So he developed a rhythm of sleep and wakefulness. By will power he stayed awake for a greater part of his day.

EDISON'S SLEEP HABITS

Thomas Edison, more than any other man, changed twentieth century *homo sapiens* from an early-to-bedder to a late-stay-upper. His little electric light bulb did that. Those who shed darkness by the kerosene or the gasoline lamp—or by candle—went to bed much earlier than we. Why? There was nothing else to do.

Who knows but that the compulsion behind Edison's discoveries was to keep the rest of the human race awake because his own life was one of wakefulness.

According to George Sands Bryan, "Edison was constitutionally able to get along with relatively little sleep. . . . In Boston he devoted from 18–20 hours to his job, his reading, and his special experimenting."

Dyer and Martin wrote that when Edison was in Newark,

> half an hour of sleep three or four times in the 24 hours was all he needed. . . . At West Orange in 1888, while developing the wax-cylinder type of phonograph, he put in five days and nights of continuous work, and this remained his record performance.

In 1920 T.C. Martin wrote: "Edison sleeps well at 73. When he sleeps he does nothing else. He never dreams, nor is he restless. He seems to have the faculty of getting more rest out of two hours than most men get out of six or eight."

Once Edison had been working around the clock and didn't get to bed until about five in the morning. He was up at seven, having had less than two hours sleep. At breakfast he said he would be feeling better that morning had he not overslept by half an hour. He felt that lack of sleep never hurt anybody.

Many people say that their sleep habits depend on their job requirements. Says one: "If I didn't have to be at the office so early, I'd probably sleep at least eleven to twelve hours every night."

That may seem like a comforting thought, yet one wonders if he would sleep that long. According to many studies, the body is usually satisfied with eight or nine hours' sleep nightly. This was shown, for example, when members of the British North Greenland Expedition (twenty-five men were away one to two years at a base less than eight hundred miles from the north pole) were permitted to sleep at any time during the twenty-four-hour nights of Arctic winter. The expedition members averaged 7.9 hours of sleep a day even though they were at liberty to sleep as long as they liked.*

THERE IS NO BLANKET FORMULA

Remember these findings, you whose jobs catapult you into the world mornings long before you have a mind to surrender your bed. Forget the millennium that will allow you to stay in bed as long as you like to sleep many hours of the day away. Chances are you'd hop out of bed after eight (or 7.9) hours sleep, wide-eyed and ready to take an active part in living.

* These findings were reported to the British Association for the Advancement of Science meeting in Sheffield, England, by Drs. H.E. Lewis and J.P. Masterton of the Medical Research Council, Hampstead, London.

For example, a man living in the country who thinks he needs at least nine to ten hours sleep goes to the city to live, and because of all the excitement he finds he needs only six to seven hours. This may be especially true if the man is in the eighteen- to twenty-five-year age group. According to some researchers, men in this age group need less sleep (six to seven hours) than those in any other age level. Much will depend on physical and emotional makeup: the lean, overactive type sleeps irregularly; the pyknic, or squat, type sleeps deeply and well. If he is a manual worker, he will require more sleep than the so-called brain worker. But I must stress that there is no overall formula that will serve us all. Many people in excellent health sleep only five hours nightly.

EACH HAS HIS OWN SLEEP RHYTHM

As I've already said, one individual reaches his peak minutes after rising, another not until noon and a third not until late in the day. In my experience in dealing with patients, this variance is often the cause of many husband-wife arguments. Physiologically, their gears do not mesh. It's the old story of oil and water.

For example, Mr. Smith comes in to breakfast, lids still drooping and half-asleep. His wife, one of the early-morning types, asks him about the international situation or whether he doesn't think the living room should be painted, or about the trip to Switzerland he mentioned at the party last night. Smith looks at her befoggedly, sees nothing more than an outline in the space opposite him and grunts. More often he shouts, and they are off to the races in an altercation.

Or, a wide-awake husband will make a simple request for

a clean handkerchief or ask about last month's electric light bill, and his stuporous wife ("dead to the world until I can have my coffee in the morning") will turn on him suddenly like an enraged lioness.

Slow wakers don't make for pleasant company. Many take two hours to wake up fully. It's too bad, but fast wakers are a much rarer breed than slow wakers.

Sir Winston Churchill once said that he attributed the success of his marriage to the fact that he breakfasted only once with his wife during all the years of their marriage. Whatever the reason, or method, the Churchills overcame early morning incompatibility. Is there anyone who really feels fine on waking? It's just a matter of who gets over this early morning depression more quickly.

We are brightest when the body temperature is highest. Even so, peak efficiency lasts only about two hours. Some don't reach their peak until as late as 11 P.M. (probably you have seen them at parties; they don't want to go home). It has been said that very bright people need little sleep, but I have heard dunces prattle about how little sleep they required.

DETERMINE YOUR OWN SLEEP REQUIREMENTS

Many husbands and wives are unhappy with each other because of a difference more in temperature than in temperament. It is important for each one of us, married or not, to determine where we fit in. Are we really night owls or early birds?

Take your temperature every hour during the day for a few days. Write down the readings. Keep a temperature chart. See if the daily lows and highs coincide. Remember that you are at your best during higher temperatures. You may be able to rearrange your work and home schedules for greater efficiency. The early bird has a higher temperature in the morning; the reverse is true for the night owl. Temperature cycles differ. Some fortunate people fit into either category. They adjust easily to work and people. A complementary sleep rhythm is so important to marriage that every married person should know his category. Job-wise and marriage-wise, temperature readings may be more important to you than you realize. Try the thermometer test for a few days.

CHILDREN'S SLEEP NEEDS VARY, TOO

It is generally accepted that infants under one month need twenty-one to twenty-three hours of sleep a day; a six- to eight-year-old child requires twelve hours; a boy or girl of thirteen to fifteen needs nine to ten hours; and the average adult needs eight hours.

However, just as there is no "average" yardstick applicable to every individual, so it is true that we differ in our sleep requirements as much as we do in height and other characteristics.

Too often we forget that children are small adults. (Some would rather say that adults are large children.) Whichever way you prefer, the fact remains that sleep is purely personal. Some children, like some adults, require less sleep. It is these children who cause their parents so much grief because they do not get as much sleep as the neighbor's children.

Like some men and women, some children are born night owls. They are not being persnickety, stubborn or difficult when they won't go to bed at a "reasonable" hour. All they are being is themselves. They just aren't sleepy. How would you react if someone insisted in tucking you in at 9 or 10 P.M. when you were wide-awake and wanting to be up and doing?

And so the children kick and scream; they use subterfuges such as thirst, pain and scores of other well-known tricks to wear down the parents until they say, "Oh, all right. But remember now, you can only stay up for another half-hour." And the child hops out of bed as if relieved from shackles and heavy chains.

I recall one mother who was distracted because her youngster, a girl aged four, slept only eight hours nightly and hadn't napped since the age of fourteen months. She couldn't understand that her little girl was a night owl by nature, and that it would be better to accept the fact than to fight it and become obsessed about it.

Baude has said that insomnia is "a contagious disease often transmitted from babies to parents." How true. If mothers would only realize that it isn't true that every infant needs twenty to twenty-two hours sleep every night, they would be happier. Doctors should remind them that the majority may even do well on only fifteen hours of sleep, and that this is even true for some babies who are only two or three weeks old.

PARENTS WORRY TOO MUCH ABOUT CHILD'S SLEEP

But young mothers will find something to worry about, especially with their first baby—and who is to blame them? I recall one woman who was certain that her baby wasn't getting sufficient restful sleep because the little fellow slept with clenched fists. The fact is that babies commonly sleep that way. They are as relaxed with clenched fists as with fingers spread out.

Is it any wonder that the newborn child is a jailer for loving parents, even though he be a welcome jailer? And the grown child remains forever the infant in the eyes of his loving parent. When he is young, he has a way of getting you up; and when he gets older, he has a way of getting you down.

Who hasn't worried about adolescents out late at night? We are concerned, not only that they may be in an accident, but also with the ever present thought that their growing bodies are being deprived of necessary sleep. How will they grow? Will loss of sleep affect their minds? Will they come down with some terrible disease because they are run-down?

So go the parental thoughts—one galloping over the next—as they lie in bed waiting for the key to turn in the lock. The answer is that the night owls can keep it up and the early birds will soon cry "Enough!"

SLEEP NEEDS FOR THE ELDERLY

Somehow the belief has got around that the elderly need less sleep than the middle-aged or young. I doubt that this is true. Whatever the time of life, seventy weeks or seventy years, "the average sleep requirement is no more applicable to a particular individual than an *average* size hat would be." It continues to remain a personal problem.

Oldsters who tell you that they needed eight to nine hours years ago perhaps forget that they are heavy and frequent nappers during the day. The naps take up the slack.

It is true that the restless man with prostate trouble who must rise a few times a night to urinate gets less sleep than he used to. But somewhere, somehow he will make it up if he needs it. If he doesn't, then he is an elderly night owl and not a young night owl.

I prefer not to lay down sleep rules for individuals who are just that: individuals. They will know their inherent requirements and will find ways to satisfy their bodily needs. From cradle to grave we follow our own inclinations in the rhythmic unconsciousness that prepares us for the following day. "Tell me not how much to sleep and I promise not to tell thee, either."

Jim Bishop wrote, "Me, I sleep by the clock and do pretty well. I retire at 2:30 A.M. and arise at 9:30 A.M. At 5 P.M. I sneak a nap for 30 or 40 minutes. It is half-way between a doze and a sleep, known to my children as a 'dope.' "

But Arthur Brisbane needed more. He used to say that it takes two weeks of regular sleep to overcome the shock of one night's incomplete rest.

A recent study of a small group of patients, all over sixty, was quite revealing to Dr. Philip M. Tiller, Jr., of New Orleans, Louisiana. He found that it isn't true that older persons need less sleep than younger ones. Those who had been getting less than seven hours' sleep a night complained of fatigue, tension, apprehension and many physical discomforts. These symptoms improved when their sleep quota was increased to nine to ten hours a night, plus an hour or two during the day. Sleep seems to be good medicine for the "functional illness" of the elderly. I have observed similar improvements in my own care of older patients.

Many elderly people complain bitterly of insomnia. They blame their symptoms on lack of sleep. In "A Survey of the Sleep Habits of 509 Men of Distinction," a paper written in 1931, Dr. D.A. Laird reported that the average duration of sleep in the seventh decade of life was seven hours and forty minutes, and in the ninth decade, eight hours and ten minutes.

I believe that we have accepted for too long (and without scientific proof) the theory that as the life-span increases the need for sleep decreases.

The elderly complain and cry out for sleep because they know that sleep deprivation makes them feel worse. Possibly their craving for more sleep is no more than an instinctual urge to counteract physical degeneration. Perhaps that is why they doze off so often, why they take naps—not because they are old, but because nature prods them into restoring spent nervous energy.

Rather than complacently accept the prevailing theory that the elderly require less sleep, I go along with the Russian scientist Professor Braines, whose theory is that the insomnia common as we grow older is an important factor in hastening senility. As I have told patients, "If you would stay young longer, sleep longer."

What is true for the older is certainly so for the young. In an interview Tony Conigliaro, nineteen-year-old, 6′3″, 180-pound Boston Red Sox star, said: "The more I sleep the lighter the bat feels. If I get only 11 or 12 hours, I can feel the difference. Really."

Some young mothers suffer from depression after the birth of a baby—sometimes known as the "baby blues." Lack of sleep during pregnancy, during labor and during the first few weeks after childbirth may well be the contributing factor.

When a person is deprived of sleep, the psychological upsets and disturbances are often more disabling, and appear sooner, than any physical impairments.

4 | Narcolepsy: Enemy of Insomnia

DO THEY CALL YOU SLEEPYHEAD? Is someone always after you to "wake up and get going"? Man (woman or child), you may be the innocent victim of narcolepsy. Consider this revelatory letter from a complaining wife:

> Dear Dr. Steincrohn:
>
> What have you to tell me of such a complaint as too much sleep? Is it possible to get too much? Besides causing loss of strength and energy, is it harmful?
>
> My husband is forty-five. I have watched him gradually deteriorate since television came into our house. Yet I can't say that I blame it all on TV because he has been sleepy since we were first married.
>
> He doesn't go in for strenuous exercises and doesn't exert himself much in his work. He puts in long hours but can hardly stay awake. He is accustomed to a nap nearly every day after a midday meal. He is usually home by 7:30 P.M. and is habitually undressed for bed, watching TV and asleep by 9 P.M. He lacks energy and shows little interest in anything but his work. I estimate that he rests and sleeps at least fourteen hours a day.

And here is a letter from another wife beset with the problem of living with a sleepy husband. From the tone of these two letters you can readily understand that sleepiness can be as troublesome as sleeplessness.

Dear Dr. Steincrohn:

I hope very much that you can help. My husband has been to several doctors, and they say he is in excellent health. Yet, every day when he comes home from work he reads the paper and falls asleep for two or three hours. Then, about 11 P.M., he goes to bed for good and sleeps until 7 A.M. He returns from work at 4:30 P.M., and it's the same routine all over again. If he is in such good health as the doctors say, why does he require so much sleep? He has tried every vitamin pill in the book but he's still sleepy. Not being able to stay awake is ruining his life and ours.

NARCOLEPSY OFTEN OVERLOOKED

In my practice I have observed similar problems. Often the correct diagnosis had been overlooked, and the unsuspecting patient carried around the label "lazy" or "good-for-nothing" for most of his life. Nobody, doctors included, could understand why the misunderstood victim slept so much of his life away.

Sometimes we just said that the patient was bored with life. Other times we suspected that the thyroid gland was underactive and prescribed thyroid extract. Only rarely did such treatment bring wakefulness to such unambitious, sleepy people. Not until recently has the medical profession become more aware of narcolepsy.

True narcolepsy is of unknown origin. It affects from 0.2 to 0.3 per cent of the population. This means that about half a million Americans may be labeled sleepyheads (most without even being aware that there is a medical reason for such laziness).

Many insomniacs have told me that they would give anything to be able to sleep most of the time. My answer is that they should be thankful they do not suffer from narcolepsy. It is one thing to sleep fitfully at night and another to have to struggle through every day trying to stay awake.

THE IRRESISTIBLE DESIRE TO SLEEP

Narcolepsy comes from the Greek words "narke" meaning stupor and "lepsis" meaning seizure. It sometimes runs in families. Those afflicted may fall asleep while eating or playing cards, when sitting in company or while at the wheel of a car—in fact, at any time. Do you recall the anecdote about the young soldier Lincoln pardoned for falling asleep while on guard duty? It is possible that the youngster was a narcoleptic.

The condition may develop during adolescence or in the second or third decade of life. In seven out of ten cases reported in one study narcolepsy appeared before the age of twenty-five. Males appear to outnumber females, sometimes two to one. It seems to be most prevalent among tall, heavy-set, athletic types who have become obese.

For example, one of my patients was a young man who had been an outstanding guard on his college football team. When he graduated he weighed 250 pounds; a year later he was up to 270. Meanwhile, he had developed the typical symptoms of narcolepsy. He was always drowsy. At last he turned to medical help because he was threatened with the loss of his job. With proper medication he regained his former pep and vim and successfully negotiated the long climb up the executive ladder of his company.

The irresistible desire to sleep overcomes people with narcolepsy as often as ten to fifteen times a day. They are continually fighting off the desire to sleep. A heavy meal at noon usually incapacitates them for the rest of the day.

If they have a monotonous job or have to listen to a public speaker for a long time, they drop off to sleep—sometimes for only a few seconds, but more often for at least ten to twenty minutes. Most patients feel refreshed after such long naps, but others resent being awakened because they are still weary and mentally depressed.

Although we do not know the real cause of most cases of narcolepsy, we are aware that it is sometimes a complication of other medical problems, such as encephalitis, brain tumor, meningitis, hysteria, cerebral arteriosclerosis, epilepsy, diabetes, hepatic disease and malnutrition.

For example, in one study of 775 patients who had brain tumor it was reported that 115 complained of pathological sleep. Somnolence was an outstanding symptom of their illness.

When found in children sleepiness may not be narcolepsy. Often youngsters fall asleep during the day to "escape" from unpleasant situations at home. (Many a child cries himself to sleep when he would rather be awake.)

Gelineau defined narcolepsy as a "rare neurosis characterized by an invincible need for sleep, ordinarily of short duration, occurring at longer or shorter intervals of time, often several times the same day, forcing subject to fall to the ground or to lie down in order to avoid falling."

Although it is not so common in early youth, narcolepsy may begin as early as the pre-teen years. It also occurs during the act of sexual intercourse (especially after orgasm). The scientific term "orgasmolepsy" is sleep or loss of consciousness brought on by orgasm.

SOME COMPLICATIONS OF NARCOLEPSY

There are complications or associated conditions accompanying narcolepsy. For example, consider "cataplexy," in which there is a sudden decrease in, or loss of, muscle tone. It occurs in about two-thirds of the cases of narcolepsy. Cataplectic seizures last less than a minute and rarely occur more than once a day.

According to a description of cataplexy by C.P. Wagner, "Immediately and without warning, there is a complete loss of muscle tonus. If [the patient] is standing he sinks to the ground. . . . [The] attack in no way resembles sleep. . . . [The patient] is aware of his surroundings throughout the attack and when he recovers, he does not feel as though he had slept." Throughout the attack, Wagner says, he remains conscious. And though he cannot move, he can hear what is going on.

However, in some cases it is true that consciousness is lost, and the sufferer feels he has gone through a terrifying dream. Sometimes a fit of laughter will bring on an attack of cataplexy.

How to make the diagnosis of narcolepsy? In one out of every four cases of narcolepsy the stricken one is unable to move or cry out, even though he feels awake. These symptoms last for a few seconds or minutes. It is almost the same as being awake during a nightmare but being helpless to do anything about it.

In about one out of every three cases the patient has what we call "hypnagogic hallucinations."

When the patient describes the classic symptoms, it is not difficult to diagnose narcolepsy. However, one has to be alert, because if the patient complains only of fatigue, the doctor may erroneously diagnose hypothyroidism. In many cases basal metabolic rates are borderline. When such rates are found in patients with narcolepsy, it is probable that sustained drowsiness and not a faulty thyroid is the cause of the lowered basal rate.

Whenever suspicions of narcolepsy arise and diagnosis cannot be definitely made, examination of brain waves will often suggest numerous episodes of drowsiness and thereby help in making the diagnosis. Diagnosis may also be made by means of empirical trial with such drugs as Ritalin, Benzedrine, Dexedrine and Desoxyn. If sleepiness and fatigue are due to narcolepsy, these drugs will wake up the patient and generate the energy he has lacked.

For many patients the most effective drug is Ritalin. The doctor prescribes it in divided doses to be taken one half-hour before meals. Sometimes it causes such side effects as nervousness, loss of appetite and insomnia. But I have found that when the proper dosage of this or similar drugs is instituted, at least 75 per cent of narcolepsy patients get very good relief.

LET US BE AWARE OF NARCOLEPSY

If we are aware of the possible presence of narcolepsy, we will not be likely to call some people sleepyheads and others stupid students.

Although it is true that narcolepsy can cause actual incapacity, most cases can be satisfactorily relieved by drugs, such as those mentioned. Remember that the predominant symptom is drowsiness—usually sustained in varying degrees.

If we are not careful, we will overlook the true diagnosis and give the affliction an incorrect label. Hypothyroidism is, I believe, the most common mis-diagnosis. The borderline thyroid tests throw us off the diagnostic trail in patients who complain chiefly of tiredness.

Sometimes narcolepsy patients are confused with those we call neurotics. On closer questioning it is usually found that neurotics say they are more tired and exhausted than sleepy. Besides, the narcoleptic patient awakes refreshed, while the neurotic remains tired and sleepy. In some cases narcolepsy has to be differentiated from epilepsy, encephalitis and hyperinsulinism (hypoglycemia).

In short, it is wiser not to attempt your own diagnosis of narcolepsy for a "lazy and tired" member of your family. Often diagnosis is not that simple.

I pity the adults and, more, the little children or adolescents in whom proper diagnosis has been overlooked. It hampers their school work and their acceptance as conscientious members of the family. They get pinned with the "laziness" tag, and worse.

They are forever sleepy. They can't concentrate. A good tipoff is the child who falls asleep while watching an exciting TV show. That is about as good a diagnostic test as any. Suspect narcolepsy—especially if the child falls asleep while talking, eating or reading.

When you are almost asleep at the wheel of a car, you know how distressing it is to force yourself to keep your eyes open. Your very life, and that of others, may depend upon your success in staying awake. In the same way, the very happiness and future of a child may depend upon the correct and early diagnosis of narcolepsy. Otherwise, he may stumble through life as some kind of drowsy dunce, despite having a high IQ.

A RARE TYPE OF SLEEPINESS

Another type of interference with wakefulness is described by Macdonald Critchley, M.D., of the National Hospital, London. It is a relatively rare phenomenon in which attacks occur about every six months and last about a week. (I have not observed it in my own practice.)

After a number of attacks the condition gradually disappears. It occurs in adolescents, most of whom have no history of previous neurotic or psychotic traits. This periodic somnolence may come on suddenly, sometimes preceded by a few days of fatigue and headache. The precipitating cause may have occurred a week previously: a fright, an injury or a bout of drunkenness.

The most prominent symptom is somnolence. The patient sleeps during most of the attack, waking only to take care of his usual bowel and bladder habits. If he is prevented from sleeping, he becomes irritable, slovenly and quarrelsome. Whenever he is awake, he eats extraordinarily large amounts of food.

Usually he acts confused and speaks of vivid dreams and waking fantasies. As a reaction to the attack he may suffer from headaches, depression, loss of appetite and inability to sleep. Asked about the attack after their recovery, most patients suffer from total amnesia with regard to their episode of somnolence.

A CONTINUING PROBLEM

The pleas for a "good night's sleep" go on and on. But conversely, cries for help continue to come from those who sleep too much. For example:

Dear Dr. Steincrohn:

Sleep! How come some people in the forty-five age bracket can get along on four hours' sleep while others like me need sixteen to eighteen hours a day? I get up at 5 A.M. to be at work by 7 A.M. We get a ten minute coffee-break, and I sleep for the full ten minutes.

We get a half-hour for lunch during which I eat my lunch in five minutes and sleep soundly for twenty-five minutes.

I quit work at 3 P.M. and am home by 3:15. I then lie on the couch and go sound asleep till 5 P.M. I eat supper, read the paper, do a few odd jobs and become so tired by 7:30 that I go to bed.

This goes on every day of the week. Then if I have nothing to do on Saturday, I go to bed Friday at 8 P.M., don't eat breakfast or lunch on Saturday and sleep till 5 P.M. I eat, do a few odd jobs and by 8 P.M. I am so tired I can't keep my eyes open, so go to bed again. Then I sleep till about 11 A.M. on Sunday. I eat brunch, go for a ride and hit the hay again at about 8 P.M.

I know it is not work that is making me tired. For I have been in the hospital for the past few months with two broken legs, and I need just as much sleep now as I did when I was working. Even now I sleep twenty hours out of the twenty-four.

I hate to drive a car for fear I may fall asleep at the wheel, which I have already done more than a few times. Have you a solution?

My first suggestion to him was: "Keep away from the car wheel—for your sake and others'. You have been lucky so far." Second, I advised him to see his doctor. A diagnosis of narcolepsy was made. He improved quickly under medication. The distressing urge to sleep everywhere, anywhere, anytime was harnessed and brought under control.

"It's wonderful to feel alive again," he wrote.

As in anything else, immoderation brings problems in its wake. Too much sleep is as unbearable as too little.

5 Leg Jitters: Insomnia's First Lieutenant

My legs are driving me crazy!

I dread to go to sleep. I used to sleep like a baby, but for the past year or two I have been lucky to get one good night's rest during the week. I just get settled down when one of three things happens. I get either prickly sensations all over my legs, usually below the knees; or a very nervous feeling which I call the heebie-jeebies; or cramps which just seem to lie in the calves of my legs. I am sixty-seven and otherwise reasonably healthy. Have you heard of this condition, doctor? Is there a remedy?

Thousands suffer from it for years without knowing it has the distinction of a label. From experience in observing patients with "leg jitters," formally called the Restless Leg syndrome, I agree with patients who say it is the number one ally of insomnia. For years I have stood by helplessly watching miserable—but otherwise healthy—persons kick their legs spasmodically like crazy horses trying to kick their way out of their stalls during a blazing fire. These people look up into your face asking for help as their legs fly off in all directions.

I was not told about this nightly terror in medical school, never heard about it at medical meetings or even discussed it with fellow physicians. Either they hadn't noticed it in patients' histories, or they thought it a trivial complaint. ("Most patients complain about sleep.")

REPORTS ON RESTLESS LEG SYNDROME

Therefore, it was with great satisfaction that I read an article called "Restless Leg Syndrome," written by K.A. Ekbom, M.D., of the Department of Neurology, University Hospital, Uppsala, Sweden. Here, at last, was a comprehensive study of the problem that had faced me for so many years in my practice.

I recall one long-time sufferer I began to treat about thirty years ago when he was fifty. A successful business man, he was the victim of leg jitters. Night after night, until he was utterly drained of energy, his legs kicked out involuntarily, and he felt ants and other small insects "walking along his bones."

I tried every remedy I knew without bringing him any lasting relief. I was surprised that he remained my patient for so many years in spite of my many failures to relieve him. Somehow these patients seem to realize that most doctors have been ineffectual in their treatment of this stubborn condition.

One thing I learned from this patient: insomnia doesn't kill. He is now close to eighty—apparently still healthy—and still a periodic sufferer from leg jitters.

Dr. Ekbom outlined the features of the Restless Leg syndrome as early as 1944. At that time it was almost completely ignored. "Its clinical features are simple and easily recognized," he wrote. "The syndrome is so common and causes such suffering that it should be known to every physician. The descriptions given in the textbooks are, with few exceptions, sparse and partly inaccurate."

According to M. Critchley, the oldest known description

of the condition was made in 1695 by the great clinical neurologist Thomas Willis, who wrote:

> Wherefore to some, when being a Bed they betake themselves to sleep, presently in the Arms and Leggs, Leapings and Contractions of the Tendons, and so great a Restlessness and Tossings of their Members ensue, that the diseased are no more able to sleep, than if they were in a Place of the greatest Torture.

Unfortunately, in medicine some important discoveries have to be shouted from the rooftops to be heard. Only recently has corroborative evidence elicited recognition by and action from the profession.

Over 250 years later here is a letter of mild corroboration from a modern sufferer:

> Also, have you any suggestion you might print for those of us who suffer from what we call the "High Strikes"? The only description I can give is that you suddenly find that you have to keep your legs moving—it's as though every nerve in your legs is jumping at once. It can wake you out of a deep sleep. I have even had it happen while riding in a train and have had to pace the aisles for hours. I know I am not alone in this, but no one seems to have hit upon a remedy for relief, other than "walking it off." It recurs, on and off, for weeks at a time, then months will go by with no sign of it. Whatever "it" is, I hope you have some suggestions for "its" surcease!

Patients describe their sensations in many ways. It is as if something is creeping, pulling or stretching in their legs.

The legs simply cannot keep still. There are such graphic descriptions as it feels "as if my whole leg were full of small worms" or "as if ants were running up and down my bones." Others say, "I wouldn't wish it on my worst enemy"; "It spoils my life"; "I get so hysterical I could weep."

These sensations are invariably worse in the evening and at night. They occur during a lecture or during a visit to the theater or the movies. The sufferers have to leave the most exciting performances because they can't stand the inactivity. They cannot sit still at a bridge game or at a dinner party, for they are bedevilled by legs that suddenly jerk and thrash out dangerously at unwary bystanders. They walk up and down constantly "like lost souls."

Surprisingly, the majority of such patients I have seen have been well-balanced, calm persons, not psychoneurotics as you might imagine.

For example, here is a letter from a person who is far from being a psychoneurotic:

> I have had leg jitters off and on for many years and was surprised to learn that many others suffer the same annoyance. I suppose my reaction is typical: a person with a little publicized affliction tends to consider his problem unique—especially when one's doctor says, "It's due to nerves, but I can't understand why you have it. You're not nervous."
>
> My condition appears to be related to periods of tension, which, I suppose, all normal people get once in a while. If I retire in a relaxed condition, there is no problem and sleep comes promptly. If I am not relaxed and insist

on coping with daylight affairs during the hours of darkness, twitching legs are inevitable.

I have worked out a number of procedures for obtaining relief, and their use depends upon the severity of the condition. The simplest and the one generally effective for mild cases is about ten knee-bends. Accompanied by an aspirin, this handles fairly severe attacks too. The most effective but most time-consuming procedure is a prolonged soak in a hot bath, again with or without an aspirin. Finally, and not to be underrated in its effectiveness, I use a stiff shot of the wonder drug called alcohol.

As any sufferer will tell you, the feeling of discomfort increases in intensity to a point where it is suddenly and instantly relieved by a jerk. In this respect it seems very similar to the sudden breakdown of insulation on an electrical conductor exposed to an increasing potential. The galvanic effect produced on a frog leg by the application of an electrical potential to a muscle completes the parallel.

Many readers will not have witnessed this latter experiment. Have you ever seen anyone react after getting a prankster's hotfoot? Or have you ever "almost" stepped on a snake? The sudden kicks of the legs under these trying circumstances are not any more violent, I assure you, than the uncontrollable leg excursions of the sufferer from leg jitters.

Even the most intelligent patients have difficulty in describing the symptoms—owing to the fact that the sensations are not like any known phenomenon with which comparisons may be made. (Hotfoot and snake reactions are about as good as any.)

LEG JERKS DIFFICULT TO CONTROL

All patients agree, however, on two points: (1) that as long as the sensations last, it is impossible to keep one's legs still; and (2) that, however described, it is an exceedingly unpleasant sensation—some call it "diabolical."

The creeping sensations may be present in the arms as well as in the legs, but this is less likely. Some patients' creepy, crawly feeling is accompanied by pain or aching sensations. But usually patients suffer from either one or the other. Usually, too, the discomforts appear only when the limbs are at rest. Some patients say they cannot find a peaceful moment. Rarely can they sink into an armchair and find complete relaxation; they have to jump up suddenly and walk up and down. Nevertheless, most agree that the discomforts experienced during the day aren't nearly as bad as those at night.

The sensations, crawling and creeping, begin about fifteen to thirty minutes after the patient gets into bed (sometimes earlier or later). In mild cases, there are a few kicks and the patient goes off to sleep. In moderately severe ones, the kicks may last a few hours. In very severe cases, the jumps and kicks may linger until 3–5 A.M. Then they cease, and the exhausted, emotionally drained patient at last finds some two or three hours of sleep.

When the kicking begins in severe cases, it is impossible for the patient willfully to keep his legs still. He gets up to walk round the room or sits up to massage his feet and legs. Some raid the icebox. Others sit up to knit, smoke, read—kicking all the while!

Sometimes the patient gets a false reprieve: the leg kicks stop after a few hours. But his sleep is soon disrupted by another siege, and he begins his nightly wanderings. Some, on getting to sleep at last, continue to kick in their sleep.

LEG JITTERS AN ALLY OF INSOMNIA

Is it any wonder that I call leg jitters the first lieutenant of insomnia? I have had some of these patients under close observation by nurses, and the reports have come back that the tales of these patients were not at all exaggerated: they did not sleep more than a few hours nightly.

Neither heat nor cold is specific in its effect on these people. Some say that they are more comfortable if they stick their feet and legs out from under the covers. Others pour cold water on their feet before bedtime. One man found relief in winter by walking barefoot in the snow before going to bed. On the other hand, some feel more comfortable sleeping with their socks on or with a hot water bag or a heat pad. Some like a cold shower; others a hot bath. Some raise the foot of the bed; others feel better with the head of the bed raised.

How sad it is that there is a tendency by both doctors and family members to belittle the patient's misery. He is said to be "nervous." After a while he is too ashamed to talk about his complaints. So he suffers in silence. "Keep your legs still, it's only your imagination" almost brings tears to a giant of a man who has been battling this adversary for years.

An examination of many patients by Dr. Ekbom revealed no neurological abnormalities, though some patients had a slight anemia.

Dr. Ekbom's study also revealed that the Restless Leg

syndrome appeared in some patients before the age of ten; the highest age at onset was eighty-two. Mild cases are common. The incidence in men and women was practically similar. Those who suffered from mild cases did not seek advice for the condition, for it did not inconvenience them. The moderately and very severe cases are less common, but they are not rare, either.

CAUSE UNKNOWN

The cause of restless legs is unknown. Sometimes it seems to run in families, but heredity is not a proved factor. Sometimes restless legs appears during the last third of pregnancy. but as a rule it disappears immediately after delivery. The incidence of restless legs in pregnant women sometimes runs to 10 per cent.

Whether the source of the symptoms is in the spinal cord or in the limbs themselves has not been solved. What we do know is that the condition may be aggravated by anemia. When this is present, the patient often improves when he has taken iron for some weeks.

VARIOUS REMEDIES TRIED

When no proper diagnosis can be made, patients are given vasodilator drugs for at least a month. Drugs such as Priscoline, Ronical and Carbachol may help eliminate the creeping sensations in two out of three patients. It is advisable to alternate medications when there is no improvement, because one may be effective when another is of no value.

In some patients I have found that dissolving a nitroglycerine tablet under the tongue may give relief within minutes. Other medicines tried are ascorbic acid, aldehydes, dextran. In one case a unilateral lumbar sympathectomy was performed, but the creeping sensations continued unabated.

If none of the above remedies is efficacious, then it is necessary to reach deeper into the bag of tricks. The use of narcotics should be avoided, although codeine may be tried for a while. Most patients who have taken tranquilizers or sleeping pills to dull the discomforts have complained that they had to get up and walk around anyway, and that their plight was worse because the effect of the drugs made them stumble about.

MANY CASES IN MY PRACTICE

Although I have not made a detailed study of leg jitters, I have observed many cases in my own practice. I fully agree with Dr. Ekbom that leg jitters is a condition that deserves the sympathy of and the most serious investigation by the medical profession. It is not to be laughed off as a "disease of the imagination." The afflicted suffer as can only those who lie awake night after night kicking their bedclothes (and themselves) into physical and emotional shreds.

Insomnia will never be completely conquered until we have restless legs under complete control. If you suffer from leg jitters do not hesitate to take the problem to your doctor. If he is one of those who laugh it off as a creature of your imagination or say that you are abnormally sensitive, prove your sensitivity (and good sense) by leaving him and finding a doctor who will keep experimenting and fighting to relieve you of this obnoxious disorder. It is one thing to be an insomniac; quite another not to be allowed to suffer insomnia in peace.

6 | Dreams, Nightmares, Sleepwalking, Snoring

MOST OF US are only mildly curious about our dreams, but some believe they possess the master key that fits neatly into every dream and unlocks its deeper meaning. The fact is, however—whatever self-appointed experts in dream-analysis may say—dreams are still the stuff they are made of: evanescent, mystifying, mysterious shadows.

Consider the following two letters from writers who, confused by their dreams, wish for some simple explanation of their inherent meanings.

> I am neither miserable nor happy. My husband seems more interested in his work than in anything else. Recently, I was hospitalized for a minor operation. Last night I dreamed that our house was for sale, and that the most attractive man came to look at it. We were mutually attracted, and I felt a glow of happiness and well-being. Part of the house was being repaired, for there was a great hole in one section. It was not my present home: I had never lived in it. Then war started, and there was a parade of marching rabbits or guinea pigs wearing shoes. After this our house was no longer the same. It had become a hospital. I was not sick, but I had a room there. I remarked to my new friend that though I was paying for a double room, all these people were crowded in with me. A lot of women were in the hospital beds in one room. One woman, a crackpot friend of mine, was on the floor. She

smiled and said she did not like me. I replied in a friendly way that the feeling was mutual. The man was with me all the time. He was no one I know, but he said he was the husband of one of my friends. All this time my husband was in the background, and I had the idea he would not care about my new friend.

Mrs. S. writes:

> I am thirty years old, happily married for three years, and have a one and one-half-year-old baby. I have dreamed at night since I was little, but for the past two years I have dreamed every single night, all night through. The dreams are mixed: good, bad, some about friends, relatives, etc. Sometimes I remember them; other times I don't. I am exhausted when I wake up in the morning. Even when I snatch a nap during the day for an hour or so, I dream. Is there any reason or solution?

If I considered myself an expert in dream interpretation, I suppose I could come up with pat explanations. But I am not. And my guess is that six experts would arrive at six dissimilar interpretations, for there are so many theories.

There are, for example, common, if not necessarily scientific, beliefs about the symbols people often encounter in dreams: a queen or a teacher symbolizes female authority or mother love; a church, purity; food, happiness and security; climbing, ambition or potency; money, love; fire, passionate emotions; snake, gun, pole or sword, male genitals; a building, woman; cows or ocean, mother.

Then to Sigmund Freud the dream represents the disguised fulfillment of an unsatisfied longing, a suppressed wish. Thus he said: "Obviously, the dream is the life of the mind during sleep." Other experts say a dream is an unexpressed wish. Andre Tridon, for example, wrote that the "real mission of sleep is to free the unconscious, to relieve the tension due to repressions and to give absolutely free play to the organic activities which build up the individual."

In the speculative and philosophical realm, G.W. Leibniz wrote: "It is not impossible, metaphysically speaking, that there may be a dream continuous and lasting like the life of man." And in *Human Knowledge*, Bertrand Russell put it this way: "It is obviously possible that what we call waking life may be only an unusually persistent and recurring nightmare."

But because theories abound, we must come back to firm ground for a few facts and scientific truths about dreaming.

SCIENTIFIC FACTS ABOUT DREAMS

Kleitman's measurements of rapid eye movement periods —the movements may be horizontal, vertical or mixed—indicate that early in the night the dream periods are eight minutes long, and that with the passage of time they progressively increase to sixteen, twenty-two and finally twenty-four minutes. In fact, dreams vary from two seconds to thirty minutes. They do not always happen "in a flash."

Dreaming does not impair sleep. We dream more than we realize because often we do not recall our dreams. Everyone dreams for approximately 20 per cent of the sleep period: for about an hour and a half in an eight hour sleep. Dreaming occurs in the lightest stage of sleep—a fact determined scientifically by observing rapid eye movements and by taking brain-wave readings.

There is no specific relationship between what you eat and what you dream. Some of my patients were certain they dreamed more on an empty stomach; others were just as sure that their disturbed sleep was due to their eating a heavy meal shortly before retiring.

In a recent report, "Effect of a Bedtime Snack on Sleep," the authors, Drs. Lyle H. Hamilton, Robert Callahan and Frances P. Kelly, stated that "a 275-calorie snack of ready-to-eat cereal, sugar, and milk at bedtime had no statistically significant effect on the pattern of sleep, the frequency of body movement, or the subject evaluation of the night's sleep by those participating in the study."

George Mann compared the dreamer to a spectator at a theater. Before the curtain goes up on our dream-play, we twist about, trying to settle comfortably in our beds. "Then the show begins. The story holds us and we sit spellbound and quiet, except for our eyes which follow action. As the curtain falls (the dream ends) the eyes stop moving. We begin stirring again; the dream episode is finished."

Observations indicate that many animals, such as the horse, the cow and the dog, dream. And some children begin to dream when they are only two or three years old.

Though everyone dreams, not everyone dreams an equal amount. Women dream more often than men, and the unmarried more often than the married. It is said that the artistically talented dream the most. (But don't congratulate yourself. The same is said of idiots, criminals and psychopaths!)

It is uncommon to "hear" speech in dreams, and when speech occurs, it is usually the dreamer who does the speaking. Each episode in your dream takes as long to unfold as it would during wakefulness. Finally, genuinely deep sleep is dreamless.

DOCTORS AND DREAMS

During a discussion, Dr. John M. Murray, Professor of Clinical Psychiatry, Boston University School of Medicine, said that the cursory analysis of dreams was a dangerous practice. The interpretation of the symbolic meaning of a dream, particularly in the analytic situation, requires a lot of background facts and long association with the patient, he maintains. If you merely seize on one dream at random and begin to interpret it, your findings will probably be untrue. Dreams are interesting and important, but proper analysis requires time, experience and an intimate knowledge of the patient and his history. You can't just pull one out of the hat and interpret it. It is almost impossible to pick out the meaning of a dream and throw that at your patient.

Nevertheless, in his book *Psychotherapy*, Charles Berg, M.D., writes: "Even if one's opportunity of seeing the patient and understanding his problem is going to be limited to only a few sessions it is often worthwhile spending at least some of them in an attempt to analyze his dream material."

Indeed, Drs. O. Spurgeon English and G.H. Pearson, the authors of *Emotional Problems of Living*, say:

> The interpretation of dreams forms an important part of psychoanalysis and psychotherapy and is a part of the study of the human mind. Freud showed that dreams are an attempt on the part of the mind to live out its wishes and to solve its conflicts. It might also be said that dreams are

a way of revealing to the dreamer, or to the doctor, what is going on in the unconscious. Mental activity goes on all the time we are asleep.*

I do not quote the master, Freud himself, because to do so would be to get us into a discussion of dreams beyond our depth in this simple consideration of the problems of sleep. If you are interested in making a further study of dreams, you may wish to read Freud's *Interpretation of Dreams* and other authors' books on the subject.

Many experts disagree with Freud. For example, in his extremely interesting autobiography, *Incurable Physician*, Dr. Walter C. Alvarez writes:

> Freud felt that the "interpretation of dreams is the royal road to the unconscious." I cannot see how Freud could have had any certainty that what he said about a dream was true. How did he know? I wonder if two or three analysts, presented with the story of one dream, would give the same interpretation of it.**

Whom to believe? The choice is yours.

Dr. Kleitman found that people are less likely to dream if they go to bed "excited, worried, and wide-awake" or "sleepy, tired or depressed" than if they go to bed "moderately tired."

In an analysis of 381 dreams of six young women, Dr. Kleitman found that "29 per cent were pleasant, and 57 per cent unpleasant, the unpleasant emotions occurring in the following decreasing order of prominence: perplexity

* O. Spurgeon English and G.H. Pearson, *Emotional Problems of Living* (New York: W.W. Norton, 1945).

** Walter C. Alvarez, *Incurable Physician: An Autobiography* (Englewood Cliffs, N.J.: Prentice-Hall, 1963).

and hurry, discomfort and helplessness, fear, anger, disappointment, shame."

People really disturbed by dreams should consult a psychologist or a psychiatrist trained in interpretation. At least they will then have the best scientific opinion. People who have persistent and frightening dreams should not rely on "dream books" in which non-experts don the robes of oracles. Nor should they subject themselves to the well-meaning but far-out interpretations so willingly offered across the backyard fence.

DREAMS AND HEALTH

Returning to the physiological changes that occur during dreams, we learn that when a person ascends from a deeper phase of sleep to the REM stage, his closed eyes dart about restlessly, his oxygen consumption increases, his brain temperature rises and his breathing and pulse become irregular. Yet, despite this apparent excitement and actual physiological change the patient may report having had only a mild, undisturbing dream.

We have learned that both deep sleep and lighter dream sleep are essential. A person deprived of the latter, his REM sleep, exhibits obvious, deleterious changes in behavior, which disappear when he is allowed to "make up" his dream-loss on subsequent nights. His anxiousness, irritability and inability to concentrate disappear.

Little REM sleep has frequently been observed in the mentally ill, the senile and those taking large doses of barbiturates and alcohol. Continued studies of the dream state may give us invaluable clues to human behavior.

As far back as 1886 Dr. W. Robert Hamburg said that

dreams provide a safety valve for the mind: they allow accumulated daytime tensions to be discharged. He also believed that, deprived of his dreams, an individual might become mentally disturbed. And Hughlings Jackson said, "Find out about dreams and you will find out about insanity."

Let us leave the last word to the editors of the *Annals of Internal Medicine*. They hold that sleep is important as a "symptom and sign of disease." The nature of sleep, they said, often holds the clue to the quality of the patient's mental and physical health. "Dreams are the stuff of the mind, the inspiration of the genius, the terror of the superstitious, the well-spring of human mythology, the bonanza of the fortune-teller, the working material of the psychoanalyst, and—apparently—an essential component of every man's sleep."

NIGHTMARES

Sometimes doctors have a perverted sense of humor. For example, we used to laugh at people who came in complaining of hay fever; there was something clownish and funny about a patient with red nose and bleary eyes. Now we recognize this form of allergy for the enemy it is. We take it more seriously. Today, physicians often tell the patient disturbed by frequent nightmares to "forget it." But it's advice hard to follow, as these letters make clear.

Dear Dr. Steincrohn:

I am writing in the interest of my husband. He has been having terrible nightmares for the past thirty years. He will wake me up night after night with the most unholy shrieks you ever heard. I have to shout at him a few times before he comes out of it. Sometimes he has as many as three nightmares in one night.

He says he can hear me calling out to him, but he's helpless to do anything about it. I shake him real hard, and then he comes to life. What he eats doesn't seem to make any difference. He will have nightmares on milk and crackers as often as he will on a steak dinner. Can you give me some kind of advice that will help him overcome this trouble?

For years I have been bothered with nightmares. They actually seem real to me at the time. Usually I can convince myself it is only a dream and force myself to wake. This in itself is a horrible feeling. When fully awake the sensations of the nightmare are still with me and I have a terrible headache from the strain.

Is it possible for a person to lose control of his mind during a nightmare? I always have the feeling that part of my mind is slipping away from me. When my husband is away on a trip, the nightmares are worse. In the dreams someone is always trying to break into the house and kidnap the children. Right now my real worry is whether a person can lose control of his mind during a nightmare.

I am twenty years old, married, have one child and am expecting again. What I would like to know is what causes people to have the same dream more than once? I have severe nightmares, and many times they have been repeated. Some nights I wake up, and I'm afraid to go back to sleep again. My nightmares usually involve me in a very intricate murder. I know very clearly how the murder is performed. Then, because I was a witness, I dream that the killer is after me. I wake up sweating, just when I'm about to be caught. Can you shed some light on this for me? I'm beginning to dread bedtime.

The late Edward Weiss, M.D., of Philadelphia, said that "grinding teeth and nightmares are indications of tension during sleep. This may account for heart attacks at a time when it was assumed that the person was not under a strain. . . . Physical rest is not synonymous with peace of mind."

Many patients have experienced a steady downhill course seemingly related to nightly recurrences of terrible nightmares. In a few cases involving the deaths of patients with severe coronary disease and very high blood pressure, I am convinced that bad dreams were an important factor. There is little question that intense emotional excitement commonly experienced in nightmares can raise the blood pressure and heart rate to dangerous limits. (More about this in the chapter on Heart Disease.)

VARIOUS SLEEP ABNORMALITIES

There are many sleep abnormalities (dyssomnias or parasomnias): nightmares, night-terrors (children are unable to recall the experiences the following morning), somnambulism, grinding of teeth, enuresis (bedwetting), delirium and non-epileptic convulsions. However, repeated nightmares seem to be the most common and most troublesome.

In their article "Sleep Disturbances," in the *Journal of Nervous and Mental Diseases*, H.R. Weiss, Ph.D., B.H. Kasinoff, M.D., and M.A. Bailey, Ph.D., remark that "reported sleep disturbances apparently are almost exclusively emotional in origin and probably represent a state of general personality distress." Their researches indicate that sleep problems seldom result from physical distress. Thus, "psychiatric patients have a much higher proportion of sleep difficulties than do medical patients or persons with no psychiatric or medical disability," and sleep troubles also increase with "increasing age, unemployment, and lower educational and occupational status."

Nowhere in my remarks or in the scientific papers I have been discussing is there a specific remedy for nightmares. How to reduce their intensity? How to modify their occurrence? Sorry. No answer. It is not so much what you eat before bedtime as what you are that seems to influence the nature of your sleep.

CHILDREN'S NIGHTMARES

Parents are often much concerned about a child's recurring nightmares. Neither the child nor the parents can understand why he should be experiencing nightmares so often. In fact, the horrible dreams are nothing more than manifestations of anxiety, a way of reactivating some unpleasant experiences suffered previously.

Probably no child or adolescent escapes nightmares at one time or another. Only when they recur with great frequency is there reason to believe that the child is being forced to handle many frightening stimuli during the day. It is then the job of both doctor and parents to inquire into the reasons, especially since nightmares are often an indication that the child needs help with his interfamily relationships.

Perhaps the parents who think themselves loving and understanding are not giving the child a feeling of security because they do not know how to show their love. Perhaps they do not have that love. Perhaps they are actually rejecting the child. Is it any wonder that while the child is asleep, the unconscious goes to work and reenacts—in disguises—the baleful experiences the child undergoes day after day? Here, too, is sufficient reason for sleepwalking during puberty in many children whose lives are full of stress and frustration.

Bruxism (teeth grinding or gnashing), like nightmares, may indicate abnormal tensions. Probably it occurs during the dream state. It is common in both children and adults of both sexes. Studies of sleeping cats have revealed movements of jaws and whiskers coincident with REM periods, so perhaps cats suffer from a form of bruxism, too.

SLEEPWALKING

Some call it somnamubulism. Dr. J. Isador Sadger in his book *Sleepwalking and Moonwalking* calls it noctambulism and writes:

> In sleepwalking a person rises from his bed at night, apparently asleep, walks around with closed or half opened eyes, but without perceiving anything, yet performs all sorts of apparently purposeful and often quite complicated actions and gives correct answers to questions.

Dr. Sadger adds that the sleepwalker can never remember what he said or did when he awakens. But whatever it is called, sleepwalking remains a stubborn problem.

Sleepwalkers have been known to drive cars and climb trees, and later to give dream explanations for their actions. Noctambulism occurs most frequently in children before the age of puberty. Often women are no longer bothered with it after they have given birth to their first child.

Many believe that sleepwalking is a symptom of a neurosis. Thus Commander B.I. Kahn, M.C., and Lt. R.L. Jordan, M.C., of the U.S. Naval Hospital, Oakland, California, in their article in the California section in *Modern Medicine* magazine, concluded that (1) "sleepwalking is an aggressive or sexual motor activity aimed primarily at a fear-inspiring father"; (2) "the somnambulist is [usually] naive, infantile, emotionally labile, impulsive, moderately histrionic and egocentric"; (3) "the chief identification figure . . . is an authoritarian, frightening father with strong religious trends"; and (4) "the mother . . . is submissive, timid, indifferent, and ineffectual." Because the sleepwalker fears the father and cannot express resentment for the mother, he works out his suppressed feelings in sleepwalking, dreams and nightmares.

BE THANKFUL FOR GOOD SLEEP

As you can see, sleep can be all honey and it can be sour wine. People who hit the hay and rise and shine, refreshed, after an undisturbed sleep do not realize how fortunate they are. It means that they spend about one-third of their lives in complete comfort.

I sleep well as a rule, yet about nine months ago I had one frightening nightmare I shall not forget. It was so vivid and so much of a threat that I can still visualize it clearly. It is, therefore, with much sympathy that I listen to the people who beg for a remedy for the nightmares they suffer night after night.

To them I say, ask for expert medical help rather than try to overcome these problems by hit or miss means. At least the physician trained in treating sleep irregularities (usually a psychiatrist) is more likely to be successful in lessening these nightly tussles with unreality than amateur sleuths who volunteer to help you.

SNORING

Think of a snorer, and you often picture a big hulk of a man, lying on his back, emitting raucous buzzes, snorts and hisses. But little women are not exempt from the nightly raspings and gurgles that bring insomnia to their mates. At least one in eight Americans snores—as many women as men. If there are 25 million snorers in the United States, there are at least 25 million disturbed listeners to this cacophony of sound.

Many years ago a Colgate University psychologist studied the intensity of sound given off by snorers. In terms of loudness, the tick of a watch at three feet measured ten to thirty decibels; ordinary conversation, forty to sixty decibels; a pneumatic drill (at ten feet), seventy to ninety decibels. One group of snorers emitted snorts in the forty decibel range; another reached sixty-nine decibels. Is it any wonder, then, that I have received hundreds of letters similar to the following:

> I have the bad habit of snoring. I guess as soon as I go to bed I start to snore. It even seems that I snore when I think I am awake (so they tell me). This is getting very embarrassing. It makes me nervous because my husband needs his sleep and doesn't get it. I try so hard not to snore that I just can't lie still. I don't get my rest; neither does my husband.

> I am one of those female snorers. When I was very little, my mother was very embarrassed because I would

fall asleep in the evening church service and snore quite audibly. All my life (over a half-century) I have been kidded about this. I am sure there are many other women (as well as men) who suffer embarrassment from snoring. Won't you please offer some down-to-earth advice on how to overcome this affliction?

Air currents, as they flow over the tissues of the soft palate, cause it to vibrate and produce snoring sounds, just as a breeze causes a flag to flutter on a pole. Snoring can be produced or aggravated by a deviated septum, turbinates swollen owing to allergy or infection, polyps, large tonsils or adenoids, jaw malformations, colds, hay fever, and other such ailments.

Depending on the indications, either medicine or surgery may help the stubborn case. Antihistamines, steroid hormones or antibacterial drugs given to overcome congestion and infection often help, as may removal of polyps, adenoids, tonsils or other offenders amenable to surgical treatment.

According to the late Noah D. Fabricant, M.D.:

> Paradoxically enough, not all mouth breathers snore. However, too much smoking, overwork, fatigue, obesity and poor general health may lower the tone of the throat tissues and cause snoring.
>
> Snore for snore, the largest group of offenders are the elderly because they lack tissue tone.

At least three hundred snore-curtailing devices have been issued by the U.S. patent office. This alone indicates how ineffectual is our specific treatment. Nevertheless, we must keep on trying. For the sake of others, the afflicted should continue to try professional means to overcome his snoring.

7 | Some Common Causes of Insomnia

YOUNGSTERS WONDER WHAT YOU MEAN when you ask them if they sleep well. "Of course I do," they say. "Is there any other way?" Absence of chronic fatigue, voracious appetite, good bowel movements and "sleeping like a log" are some of the common attributes of youthfulness. Comes middle age, and later, and loss of appetite, tiredness, constipation and insomnia become more common.

Insomnia is often the most stubborn of these complaints. If you haven't been sleeping well, you belong to one of two main classifications.

Members of the first group fall asleep quickly and easily. They sleep soundly until 4 or 5 A.M., then are "wide-awake" for the two or three remaining hours before daylight. The twisting, turning and trying to sleep tire them out; they feel as though they hadn't slept at all.

Members of the second group can't seem to get to sleep. They go to bed at 10 P.M. and are still wide-awake at 1 or 2 A.M. They can't seem to let go. An unending parade of thoughts jiggle and jaggle their brains and keep them functioning overtime. Members of this group, too, awake tired and unrefreshed. They do not feel that the few hours' sleep they've had have done them good. They struggle through the next workday as if they had been carousing all night.

There are 1001 varieties of insomnia. Each seems to have a separate cause, but all insomniacs are rightfully unhappy about it all. The man or woman who works hard all day longs for rest and forgetfulness at night. Otherwise, he faces the next day (and night) with trepidation sometimes bordering on hysteria. Fatigue builds up. Few things demoralize us so much as the cumulative effects of steadily recurring insomnia.

Illness is almost a sure cause of sleeplessness. The man who is tossed by fever or wracked by pain is not surprised by his inability to sleep. The man with prostate trouble soon learns to accept the frequent trips to the bathroom that upset his sleep rhythm, as does the woman with unusually severe hot flashes that temporarily disturb her rest at night.

But how about the man who is apparently well? "I can't understand it," he says. "The only complaint I have is that I can't sleep well. It began about three months ago and seems to be getting worse. I'm not worried about business or finances. Everything is all right with my family. My wife and I are happy. Why should I stay awake for hours, night after night, thinking about *everything?* I can't seem to turn off my thoughts."

Each case of insomnia is a problem peculiar to itself. The doctor needs to question each patient carefully, and the patient must answer fully and in detail. Somewhere there may be a clue.

My own experience with patients has led me to believe that the following are some of the common reasons for insomnia: overwork (you think you leave your work at the office, but you take it home with you—in your head if not in your briefcase); chronic fatigue (which you attribute simply to loss of pep); insufficient relaxation (you think you are relaxing in bed; in fact, you are tied up in a bundle of muscular and nervous tension knots); sleeping with "one ear and one eye open" (because of concern for your children); exposure to many outside noises (which you have taken as a matter of course); too many or too few bedclothes.

Perhaps you have become a poor sleeper because your husband (or wife) tosses or turns too much in your double bed. Perhaps the coffee, tea, milk or light snack you have recently begun to take before retiring has upset the sleep balance. Perhaps one of you snores. Are you worried that you will give offense by suggesting another room to sleep in? Whatever the cause, it must be found and removed.

Long, patient talks with the insomniac are essential in order to determine the reason for his sleeplessness.

Is he justifiably concerned about his health? Or are his complaints rooted in a neurotic pattern? Is he suffering grief? Recent bereavement? Financial difficulties? Job problems tied in with unyielding interpersonal relationships?

Even worse, is the wakefulness the result of an ever-present chronic anxiety of the free-floating variety, in which there is no apparent reason for feeling threatened by the environment?

Will simple measures—such as neutralizing pain, indigestion, cough or urinary disturbances—overcome the insomnia? Does itching keep the patient awake? Hunger? Thirst? Extremes of heat or cold?

The causes of insomnia may be divided into physical and psychic factors. Transitory physical causes such as pain or poor sleeping conditions, for example, may be overcome, and the insomnia cured. But the chronic physical factors such as cerebral arteriosclerosis, chronic cough, prostate trouble, chronic pain resist treatment.

Transitory psychic factors such as tensions, anxiety, grief and strain are often easily overcome. But lasting insomnia results when psychic factors become chronic, as, for example, in those people who are in a deep depression or have morbid anxieties.

Quite often "simple" day-to-day problems interfere temporarily with night-to-night sleep. Are you anxiously waiting for a child or grandchild to be born? Are you excited over a new job? Have you just lost (or come into) a fortune? Are you down with a virus infection or plagued with headaches? Are you "remaking" the speech you made the previous evening?

Such are the transitory insomniacs. An occasional night of sleep disturbed is but a temporary island of discomfort; it does no actual harm. It is, in fact, the chronic insomniac who really suffers.

In *Our Human Body* Robert Coughlan writes: "Insomnia has never killed anyone. But to the people who suffer from it, insomnia is as debilitating as anemia, as nagging as an ulcer, as uncomfortable as a leg in a cast."

This letter about a seventy-three-year-old woman indicates clearly that insomnia "doesn't kill anyone" however long it lasts.

Dear Dr. Steincrohn:

I am writing to you to ask for your comments as to my wife's inability to get a good night's sleep. This is something that has been going on for many, many years. She is seventy-three years old and has always been sympathetic, perhaps too much so for her own good, over the troubles of others, especially those close to her.

She has two daughters by a previous marriage and has always been at their beck and call whenever she thought they needed her. She is a chronic worrier and most of the things she worries about never occur. She has been to two different doctors, and each has given her a thorough examination and found nothing wrong with her physically. They said her condition was the result of tension and worry and prescribed mild sedatives. Nothing seems to help. She takes hot baths, exercises, uses a massage pad with heat, but she still gets only three or four hours of sleep a night with few exceptions.

She goes to bed about 10:30 P.M. and gets up in the morning about 7:45 A.M., but between those hours she may awaken at 1:30 or 2 A.M. to go to the bathroom. Then when she goes back to bed, she cannot go to sleep. She tosses and turns and touches her toes and finally gets up again and goes to the kitchen and makes herself some warm milk. And so it goes.

What do you think can be done? She sleeps alone in a big double bed, and the room is quiet and dark. I sleep in a double bed at the other end of the house. We both hope you can give us some suggestions that will help.

The next letter clearly refers to the cause of the insomnia, but the sufferer refuses to take the "cure" because he will not consider seeking refuge in another room.

My wife's sinus trouble has made her very unreasonable: she claims that she has to close the bedroom windows tight, even in hot, dry weather with ninety-degree heat. Our bed is located in the hottest corner of the room, and she sleeps with her head in the corner so she won't get any air from the two windows in the room. But she allows me to open all the other windows in the house. Surely this is inconsistent? In any case, does anyone with sinus trouble need to go to such extremes? In hot weather, too?

Couldn't she open the windows a few inches without doing herself harm? I am at my wits' end and will do anything within my means to obtain a cure for her sinus trouble. But I sometimes think that keeping the bedroom airless has become a compulsive neurosis with her.

I am losing too much sleep and receive little or no comfort from retiring at night. Please do not suggest that I sleep in the other bedroom. The marriage contract implicitly requires that married couples occupy the same bedroom and the same bed. And I intend to abide by it.

TOGETHERNESS AND INSOMNIA

This last letter shows that marital relations can cause insomnia. Husbands and wives must reach mutually acceptable decisions about bedroom comfort: whether to keep the air conditioning on in summer, the heat on in winter, the windows open or closed. Then it is important to review the state of togetherness. Is there too much at night? Does sleeping in separate beds make the difference between a good night's sleep and a recurring nightly battle with insomnia?

Consider these opinions on togetherness in Dr. Elizabeth Blackwell's *Laws of Life*, written in 1852 (forgetting she is a physician, remember that this is a woman's point of view):

> There is nothing that will so derange the nervous system of a person who is eliminative in nervous force, as to lie all night in a bed with another person who is absorbent in nervous force. The absorber will go to sleep and rest all night; while the eliminator will be tumbling and tossing, restless and nervous, and wake up in the morning, fretful, peevish, fault-finding and discouraged. No two persons, no matter who they are, should habitually sleep

together. One will thrive, and the other will lose. This is the law, and in married life it is defied almost universally.

If you think this is a prejudicial, female attitude, then consider these words from a man, Dr. E.B. Foote, written in 1870:

> Married people make a great mistake in allowing themselves to sleep together. This practice, in a measure, leads to uncongeniality. From five to eight hours bodily contact in every 24, with one person, not only causes an equalization of those magnetic elements which, when diverse in quantity and quality, produce physical attraction and passional love, but it promotes uncongeniality by making the pair grow physically alike. . . .
>
> A reform in this custom, however, can hardly be expected to be made in one generation. Husbands and wives who have been in the practice of sleeping together for five or thirty years, will hardly be persuaded to relinquish the social luxury of spending their nights together, especially if their matrimonial life has led to a fair amount of social enjoyment.

FRANKNESS BETWEEN HUSBAND AND WIFE

Undoubtedly, a frequent cause of insomnia is too much togetherness in the bedroom.

A young married woman I had known since she was a little girl came to me and slumped in a chair. Her lids came down low over her eyes, and she seemed half asleep as she sat there.

"I dislike butting into your day like this," she said. "Too many of your patients need real help for serious illness. But this is serious, too. So serious I don't dare face another long night of sleeplessness. I've simply got to get some rest, and right away! The reason I've put it off until now is because Bill is so sensitive. I don't want to hurt him.

"My trouble is that I've always been a light sleeper. For the two years we've been married we've had a double bed. Bill twists and turns all night. Besides, he's a champion snorer. I know the answer is twin beds. But if I make the suggestion, I know what he will think. He won't say it, but he will question my love for him.

"Please don't laugh this off. Please promise me you will help me. I'm so tired and nervous for lack of sleep I can't go on much longer."

I have seen too much of this problem to treat it as a joke. I told her I would ask her husband to come to the office. He was a nice, open-minded young man. He admitted that he had been worried lately about her. She seemed to him rundown, tired and irritable. He did not suspect he was the innocent cause.

As tactfully as I could, I explained the problem. "Be thankful," I said, "that the solution is in your own hands, and that it is an easy one. Turn in your double bed for twin beds. There's no law that says you can't keep them close together."

His first reaction was the usual one. "Poor kid," he said. "Why didn't she tell me? Besides, I have a confession to make. I haven't been sleeping too well myself lately."

Within a week after the furniture exchange, our young lady was again filled with her usual vigor and energy.

I wonder how many readers are in a similar predicament? You can benefit from the advice I gave this young couple.

Some say that a double bed is a guarantee of married bliss, a sure bulwark against divorce. Twin beds, they say, are a psychological as well as physical step toward separation. I haven't studied the relationship between divorce and the sale of twin beds, but I doubt that happy husband-wife relationships are dependent on double beds. It's the people that count!

If I were asked to guess, I'd say there is more likelihood of loss of sleep and consequent irritability and argument in double beds than in twin beds (no elbows in the ribs, no twisting and turning). Sometimes (in the case of snoring)—or where temperature adjustments are out of mutual kilter—"his" and "her" bedrooms are the answer for keeping romance alive.

If you have been tired and irritable lately, examine your sleeping habits closely—not only how many hours you reserve for sleeping, but all ancillary conditions effective in helping or disturbing sleep.

CHECKPOINTS FOR SLEEPING COMFORT

Whether we like it or not, we are destined to spend approximately one-third of our lives in bed. Yet in many homes the bed is the least respected article of furniture. Unreasoningly, we often live a great part of our lives in unnecessary discomfort.

In homes where kitchen utensils glitter, dining room chairs and table shine and armchairs invite one to sit down in luxurious splendor, I have seen beds in which only a masochist could find comfort.

Either they were antiques, long on reputation and short on comfort, or they were too short, or they had ancient, bumpy, lumpy mattresses and springs that had been sprung years before.

I am sure it is not penuriousness that is the reason: I

blame it on procrastination. "Let's get the new refrigerator first," says the lady of the house, "there's time enough to get new mattresses."

There are many ways of "being good to yourself." You can go on a vacation; you can buy some new clothes; you can go out and buy yourself a set of golf clubs or a new car. But above all these I rate sleeping on a comfortable bed and mattress and getting a good night's sleep.

If the mattress is of ancient vintage but "still comfortable," don't think you don't need a new one. Like a twenty-year-old car, it will serve its basic purpose. But what I am talking about is up-to-date comfort and not just serviceability. There is a difference between ordinary sleep and a good night's sleep, so go shopping for a good mattress.

Take a good, unbiased look at your present mattress. Padding and binding have a way of wearing out. Is the stitching broken? Do the borders sag? Is there an odor? Can you see or feel any lumps? If so, better go shopping. Mattresses of a recent model are a necessity, not a luxury.

You will have many choices, depending on your own likes and dislikes. The usual types of mattress are inner-spring, solid upholstered and foam. The inner-spring mattress is more popular than the foam by about ten to one. It has strong coil springs of steel with insulating material and padding on both sides of the coil unit, all enclosed in a cover. Solid upholstered mattresses are stuffed with varied materials such as cotton, cattle-tail hair, horse hair and hog hair. When combined with spring action, even this kind of mattress is resilient.

Foam mattresses are made mainly from the milk of rubber trees or from synthetics. Some say the foam mattresses are too warm in summer; others prefer them, summer and winter. A good quality foam mattress made from latex is quite expensive and brings comfort when set on a good spring foundation.

For comfort a mattress should be at least eight to ten inches longer than the person's height and ten inches wider than his circumference at the waistline. Most people are more comfortable with hard mattresses that do not "give" too much. Some people with bad backs find it even more comfortable if the mattress is reinforced by a board between it and the springs.

If you are allergic, make certain that your mattress is not stuffed with kapok fiber, which may cause or aggravate your allergy. (Have you cleaned, vacuumed and aired your mattress recently? A routine monthly cleaning is the enemy of dust.) I recall one patient who wheezed and coughed, especially when she went to sleep. After many X rays and pints of cough mixture, a wily, detective-oriented allergist decided to examine her bedroom equipment. He found a kapok mattress and asked her to get another kind. Her cough disappeared within a week.

PILLOWS

How about your pillow? I tell people that the pillow, too, is an individual matter that only they can decide. Some prefer to sleep flat; others use one, two or even three pillows. Whether you prefer pillows made from feathers, horse hair or down (or of any other material) will depend on individual preferences; after all, pillows only fill the space between head and shoulders. But remember: if you are allergic, be careful to check the pillow as a possible cause of restless nights.

Many prefer a pillow that is a mixture of down and waterfowl feathers because it is more buoyant and lasts longer. Others like the less expensive combinations of chicken and turkey feathers, which make firmer pillows. If you prefer a very firm pillow go shopping for one made of synthetic fibers and hair.

BEDSPRINGS

There are three main types of bedsprings on the market: flat bed springs, metal coil springs and box springs. A patient who manufactures bedsprings insists that there is little choice where a mattress and bedspring are involved. He believes that the inner-spring mattress, which will last longer if you turn it over periodically, on a box spring is the best arrangement.

BLANKETS

The proper choice of blankets is a factor in overcoming insomnia. Remember that if you prefer a heavy covering at night, it is better to use two light blankets than one heavy one. The air cushion between two blankets helps protect against the cold. Be sure they are not too heavy. In one night your chest does quite a few thousand push-ups; multiply each chest excursion by a few extra ounces and you have jostled an unnecessary poundage.

Some people prefer 100 per cent wool blankets; others use synthetics such as Orlon, or a mixture of the two. Synthetic blankets last longer. Electric blankets? Devotees say they are the greatest invention of the twentieth century. If they're not the greatest, to me they nearly are!

SHEETS

Most women know the basic requirements for sheets. Muslin sheets with 140–150 threads per square inch are the most durable. Percale is smoother and lighter than muslin but does not last as long. I tell people, especially those with big feet, to loosen the sheet at the foot of the bed. Many do not realize that their restlessness at night is due to the feeling of being imprisoned by the tucked-in sheet. Feet need a sense of freedom. If they don't get it, then the rest of the body becomes resentful too.

Ben Franklin recommended the use of at least two beds for insomniacs. But how many beds you have is not so important as the condition of your sleeping equipment. That has to be serviceable and in order if you expect to overcome insomnia. Spend as much time in outfitting your bedroom as you do your new car, and you will have a smoother ride into the valley of sleep. Otherwise you will suffer the bumpy sleep of the insomniac. If you have ever traveled that road, you will understand what I mean.

8 | Serendipity and Sleep

SLEEP CAN BE COURTED most successfully by use of apparent unconcern. Manifest interest in conquest can result in complete denial, rejection and defeat. The harder you try to overcome insomnia, the more likely you are to fail. There is another way, and perhaps serendipity is the answer.

Serendipity. What does it mean? You will not find an adequate definition in every dictionary. Nevertheless, the word is gradually and surely finding its way into our language. And you should be able to guess one facet of its meaning by reading the following medical anecdote.

Most people know that insulin is a lifesaver for diabetic patients. But how did the Canadian investigators, Drs. Banting and Best, know that the pancreas is the source of a sugar-regulating mechanism? By using the discoveries made by earlier investigators.

In this case, the investigators were Von Mehring and Minkowski, who, intent on some experiments, made what was at the time an idle observation. They noticed that the sugar-filled urine of dogs from which they had removed the pancreas was attracting swarms of flies, but that the flies disdained the urine of dogs which still retained the pancreas. This observation led directly to the establishment of the connection between the pancreas and diabetes mellitus.

Here is an example of serendipity in action. The researchers found something valuable without looking for it—

and thereby enabled others to go on with their own experiments.

There are as many definitions of serendipity as there are interested people. For me, it means the faculty of dutifully doing your work without straining too hard to reach your objective. Success and fame are natural by-products.

Too many of us try too hard to win at cards, to discover an oil well, to succeed in business or profession, to please everyone—and we fail. Likewise, I have known many who remained ill because they tried too hard to get well.

You may wonder what serendipity, however you define it, has to do with insomnia. Perhaps you will understand when you've read this part of the little essay on serendipity written by E.P. Scarlett, M.B., of the Calgary Associate Clinic, Calgary, Alberta, Canada:

> This delightful word [serendipity], which, incidentally, I am pleased to find is coming into wider circulation, is not a creation of the aforementioned Lewis Carrol, like JABBERWOCKY.
>
> If you look up your Oxford English Dictionary you will find that it means "the faculty of making happy and unexpected discoveries by accident." . . . The word was coined by that alert bookman of the world, Horace Walpole, from the ancient name for Ceylon—Serendip, and he discovered it in 1754 in the course of reading a fairy tale called "The Three Princes of Serendip."
>
> The sentence that sparked the word read: "As their highnesses travelled they were always making discoveries, by accident or sagacity, of things which they were not in quest of." It is a most useful and delightful word, and I have forever been advocating its wider use.*

* *Archives of Internal Medicine*, III (March, 1963), 386-88.

Dr. Scarlett mentions such instances of serendipity in the course of medicine as the discovery of penicillin by Sir Alexander Fleming while he was idly observing the mold on an old bacterial plate.

Serendipity. Is it Eve with the apple or Newton with the apple? You will have to bring to the word your own definition and understanding. To quote Dr. Scarlett again, "Meanwhile we might all pray for more serendipity in this life—both within and without avenues of medicine."

Coming to the problem under consideration, here is serendipity in action against insomnia. The story is told by a patient in the Chicago area. She may not realize it, but it will not be long before she sleeps the proverbial sleep of babes.

> At forty, with classical symptoms of the menopause for over a year, I find the new experience of insomnia a real delight, a bonus, a gift.
>
> How nice to have the quiet, to think what I please without being distracted by my voluble and gregarious preschoolers and all their chums.
>
> How self-indulgent to just relax and enjoy the presence of the family without any obligations to think of their needs or desires—physical, psychological or spiritual.
>
> How pleasant if the desire for activity leads me to sew or read or write letters because I wish to and not because the tasks must be done.
>
> How luxurious to enjoy an hour or two secure in the knowledge that the doors are locked, the phone will ring only in the event of a dire emergency, that my sometimes too many neighbors won't make time demands on my sympathetic, permissive nature.
>
> Insomnia? I love it.

This woman is already on the way to recovery. Her insomnia is staggering on its last forked, diabolic legs. Unconcerned, she is giving the back of her hand to insomnia; in other words, she is allowing serendipity to take over. She will find sleep without consciously looking for it. Insomnia cannot survive in an atmosphere of total disregard.

Of all the practical pointers I shall offer you in this book to help overcome insomnia none is so important as being able to say "Nuts!" to sleep and mean it. That is real Sleepmanship. That is the only way to hit the hay.

In part two I shall discuss Sleepmanship in Illness for those who suffer the double load of sickness discomforts and insomnia. But if you are a healthy specimen, you may skip, if you wish, to part four, in which you will discover many specific, practical measures for overcoming insomnia.

Sleepmanship in Illness | II

9 | Sleep and Heart Disease

IMAGINARY HEART TROUBLE

"IMAGINARY" HEART TROUBLE is not imaginary in the sense that you have discomfort only in your imagination; I know you suffer. It is imaginary in that though you have a normal heart, you, like millions of others, experience nagging doubts about its efficiency. After all, you reason, you have all or many of the symptoms and signs of actual heart disease. Is it any wonder you have insomnia?

Take the case of a patient who has swelling of her ankles. It comes on late in the afternoon or early in the evening and disappears by morning. She thinks that the swelling is surely due to a tired heart unable to perform its necessary function of pumping blood efficiently.

Nevertheless, this patient has a normal heart. Her trouble is caused by her job. She is overweight and a saleslady. Standing practically immobile behind a counter in a department store for eight hours a day causes her ankles to swell. X rays, electrocardiograms and physical examination convince the doctor that her heart is all right. Fortunately, he can convince her, too. She is now able to sleep at night without the help of tranquilizers during the day and sleeping pills at night.

I recall the case of the 6′4″, 200-pound former football star who became deathly afraid of heart disease one night when he was awakened by rapid heart action. "My heart runs away with itself," he said. "There doesn't seem to be any reason for it, and I get almost frightened to death. Is my heart all right?"

Examination disclosed that he had what we call paroxysmal auricular tachycardia—a functional type of heart acceleration that can occur in a healthy heart. Often we do not know what causes the heart to go into high gear, but we do have ways of slowing it down so that it beats normally. Sleepless for weeks after his first attack of tachycardia, the patient required quite a bit of convincing before he really believed that his heart was normal. When he did believe, his insomnia disappeared. Anxiety and deep, refreshing sleep do not mix well.

MANY SUFFER FROM IMAGINARY HEART TROUBLE

These days, when coronary heart disease is so much discussed, most men are aware of its potential dangers. They know that chest pain is its most common symptom. Therefore, they lose sleep and actually worry themselves sick because they "just *know* it is coronary disease." They make their own diagnosis and refuse to go to the doctor because they are afraid to face the truth.

I remember one man who was sure he had coronary trouble. He had come in from a snooze in his hammock when he noticed a steadily increasing pain in his left shoulder and chest. For days he lived in quiet fear, telling no one.

At last he went to his physician. By this time the true diagnosis was evident: shingles rash had broken out on his chest. (Often an attack of herpes zoster—shingles—is preceded by pain and is not definitely recognized until the rash confirms the diagnosis.) In this case, although the shingles still made him uncomfortable, the patient said he slept for the first time in days because he was so relieved at learning it was not a coronary attack.

Like an attack of shingles, gall bladder disease, an attack of ulcer, hiatal hernia, pancreatitis, bursitis, spinal arthritis—all may simulate a coronary.

THE NURSE MAY CATCH THE DISEASE

I recall a young married woman who came in a "nervous wreck" because she hadn't slept in weeks. Why? Because she was certain she had heart disease.

"I nursed my mother for months before she died of rheumatic heart disease," she said. "One of her symptoms was shortness of breath. I have the same thing, exactly the same thing, so my heart must be bad, too. Can you blame me for losing sleep, worrying about what will happen to my three young children if I die?"

The nurse (especially if she is a member of the immediate family) frequently "catches" the disease of the patient, even though it isn't contagious. Heart disease and cancer are especially "contagious" for the anxious nurse who has been in contact with the conditions and is certain that her symptoms are similar to the sick one's.

This young woman's imaginary heart trouble was quite stubborn, as most people's are. You can't talk the patient out of his anxiety easily. You can't turn off the stream of anxiety as you can a faucet.

The woman's breathing was not the typical shortness of breath one finds in heart patients. What she had labeled shortness of breath was, in reality, frequent, sighing respiration. In the midst of conversation she would stop to take a deep breath, then she would say, "See what I mean, doctor? This is the kind of shortness of breath I've been having." At last she admitted that her mother's shortness of breath had been of an altogether different type. But not until weeks later, when she had overcome her nervous habit of taking those deep breaths, did she find peace in sleep at night.

HEART SKIPS MAY OCCUR IN NORMAL HEARTS

In like manner, many people think they have heart trouble if they have skips, which we call premature contractions or extrasystoles. Such irregular heart beats may occur in the strongest of hearts. They often come right out of nowhere: while the patient is working or while he is lying quietly in bed. And, of course, they can be frightening.

I have occasionally experienced the sensations myself, and although I know them to be of no consequence, I have had to convince myself that there's nothing to worry about. Therefore, I know that the patient needs an understanding doctor who will explain them and reassure him.

The skip, or skips, comes like a sudden thump in the chest. The heart seems to turn over in the throat. Waiting for the next heart beat to come is like waiting for the millennium: you wonder if you will be around at the time.

Normally, the doctor asks you to lower your tobacco, alcohol and food intake. But if you are not guilty of any of these excesses, all he can do is tell you to accept the fact that you do not have actual organic heart disease and prescribe special medicines to combat the skips directly. Sometimes skips disappear on this regime, never to return. On the other hand, I have known patients who have had heart skips on and off for over twenty-five years.

Insomnia compounds the confusion, fear and chronic anxiety in patients who suffer from imaginary heart trouble. Do not refuse to take pills from fear of becoming a dope fiend, because chronic sleeplessness will endanger your health and life and there is only an infinitesimal chance that you may become addicted to sleeping pills.

Nothing, however, is more important in getting a good night's sleep, and the restfulness and well-being that go with it, than accepting your doctor's pat of assurance when he says: "There's nothing wrong with your heart." There is quite a difference between heart trouble and heart disease. One is in the mind, the other in the heart itself.

CORONARY HEART DISEASE

During acute heart attacks I believe that the difference between life and death often depends on whether or not we can get the patient to sleep. Of course, in the extremely serious attack, chest pain increases and sleep becomes quite impossible.

Before we deal with the value of sleep during a heart attack, however, let us first review the nature of coronary disease. Two coronary arteries and their branches bring nourishment to the heart itself. You can understand their importance when you realize that the entire body depends on the efficient pumping-action of the heart to survive.

When the coronaries are functioning normally, they are wide enough for the bloodstream to transport oxygen and other nourishment to the tissues. You go about your business of living without even thinking of your heart, it works so effortlessly and without complaint.

But comes the time, in some people, when the coronaries

become narrowed. Not enough blood gets through to supply the needs of the heart muscle. This narrowing process is known as atherosclerosis—a form of arteriosclerosis in which cholesterol, lime salts and other substances cause the inner artery walls to degenerate, lose their elasticity and prevent the normal flow of blood.

When this process is a gradual one, the patient's first symptoms may be chest pain on exertion and excitement. Because of the constriction in his chest, he will probably have to stop to rest while walking—especially if he has recently eaten a heavy meal. We call this angina pectoris.

If the blockage (a sudden thrombus or clot formation) is sudden and abrupt, however, the blood clot shuts off completely the circulation to a portion of the heart muscle, and we say the patient is having an attack of coronary thrombosis. In the typical attack he perspires profusely, has nausea and vomiting and experiences a very severe chest pain that lasts on and off for hours; his blood pressure plummets; and his pulse becomes weak and irregular. Some such attacks are not serious at the time; others are fatal.

Complete rest for a number of weeks is imperative after an attack of coronary thrombosis to give the heart a chance to repair its circulation. Meanwhile "collateral circulation" operates, that is, the smaller arteries take over the job of the big artery blocked by a thrombus or clot.

SLEEP IS IMPORTANT

During an acute heart attack the doctor administers drugs to elevate the blood pressure, to support the heart and to prevent further clotting. But also most important is a drug to control pain and permit the patient to rest comfortably and sleep. Morphine or some similar drug removes extreme anxiety, dulls the pain and causes drowsiness, and should, therefore, not be spared. Some patients are allowed to suffer and groan during a coronary thrombosis attack because it is believed that they should not receive more than the average dose of morphine (one-quarter to one-half grain). I have given patients as much as a grain or more over a few hours to "put them under." In many serious cases I believe that this has prevented a fatality.

When the patient is struck down by a coronary of more than moderate severity, he is in shock. His eyes roll around in fear. He is as much under the influence of anxiety as he is of pain. He wonders if this is the end. Will he recover? As his eyes look up at you, the question of survival is uppermost in his mind.

The longer he is allowed to worry, the worse chance he has. You want the patient to be relaxed so no unnecessary burden will be placed on his heart, yet, as long as fear holds sway, adrenaline is being poured into his bloodstream, thus putting an added load on a sick heart by greatly increasing its rate of beating.

For this reason, therefore, it is good medicine to keep the coronary patient "under" for the first few days. Keep him unaware of what is going on: no telephone ringing; no visitors—except the immediate family (for a short while). The patient needs rest as a fish needs water. And he can't get real rest unless he sleeps. Therefore, when we ease off on morphine, Demerol and other such drugs, it is advisable to change over to tranquilizers during the day and sleeping pills at night.

VISITORS CAN BE DANGEROUS

Sometimes the coronary patient is beset by a roomful of visitors on the second or third night after his severe bout with the man with the scythe. His room is smoke-filled and noisy; visitors are sitting on the bed. You can see that only his spirit is keeping him together and preventing him from collapsing then and there.

I recall many such colossal visitor-blunders by well-meaning friends and family; with one sweep I would clear the room—no way to win friends, perhaps, but a way to save some patients.

A doctor who fights to keep his coronary patient alive is in no mood to bear damn foolishness patiently. Most people do not realize that the first ten days of what is only a mild attack are perilous. It doesn't take much to tip the scales. Visitors have unwittingly killed many a coronary patient. They send flowers a few days later, but they do not realize that the visiting session a few nights previously may have been the important factor in their friend's demise.

Sleep will do away with much of this. A patient who is asleep is not fair game for most visitors. Usually, they will turn around and go home, where they belong. If they are really concerned, they will accomplish more for the patient by sending a card or some flowers than by coming in person during the first two weeks.

Sleep, gentle sleep, is the best friend the coronary patient has. It permits complete rest and gives his injured heart muscle the opportunity to heal in peace. It is the doctor's job to help his patient sleep during those first two hectic weeks and keep visitors away. Wakefulness is the friendly cohort of dangerous complications.

HYPERTENSIVE HEART DISEASE

High blood pressure is called hypertension. Break down that word into "hyper" and "tension," and you have a fairly unobstructed view of its real meaning. The high blood pressure patient is not just tense, he is "hyper," or too, tense.

As his blood pressure climbs over the years, the continuing strain exerts a deleterious effect on the blood vessels and heart. Atherosclerosis and arteriosclerosis set in. The linings of the arteries, large and small, become crusted with limes, salts and fatty acids, the flow of blood is obstructed, the resiliency of the vessels is lessened by the loss of elasticity in the muscle walls. The big heart muscle is forced to increase its daily work to keep the blood flowing to the various cells and organs.

It is a physiological truth that when you exercise a muscle, it becomes larger. Just as isometric exercises almost guarantee a bigger biceps, so the heart, as it has to pump harder and more often than proper, also becomes enlarged. When this happens, the patient gets what we call hypertensive heart disease. The enlarged heart is usually the sick heart. Comes the time when further enlargement, necessary to accomplish its duties, exerts such a strain on the heart that it begins to fail.

The hypertensive heart patient begins to complain of shortness of breath and early fatigue. As the disease progresses, he may cough because of the collection of fluid in the lungs, his ankles may swell at night and he may find that he cannot sleep as well as he used to.

Too many hypertensive patients forget this last complaint in the shuffle of the others. This is unfortunate because sleep is often the hypertensive patient's most insistent requirement. Without sleep and relaxation all the medicines might just as well be thrown down the drain. Sleep is the base on which we build good treatment for these patients.

If you have high blood pressure and complicating heart disease, the simple remedy, such as the use of two or three pillows instead of none or one, may make the difference between a comfortable night and a restless one. Patients who are in cardiac distress are not comfortable lying flat; they have difficulty in breathing; that is, they suffer from orthopnea.

You might think that they would realize the advantage of raising their heads by trial and error, but too many don't. They go on being uncomfortable for months or years, when lifting the head of the bed or using extra pillows might well bring them more ease.

If you have hypertensive heart disease, smoking is bad for you. If you insist on taking a pipeful or an occasional cigar or cigarette, draw the line after 5 or 6 P.M. Many patients have found that not smoking in the few hours before bedtime has resulted in a good night's rest.

A drink of sherry or an ounce of hard liquor often promotes sleep when taken one half-hour before retiring. Beer is a beverage I do not advise for hypertensive patients. Some can take brandy with good effect, but others say it keeps them up by making their hearts thump.

Coffee, tea and cold drinks are not permissible. Some patients cannot even take cocoa. Hot water or hot or warm milk are the only other liquids one may take with safety.

SLEEP HELPS THE HYPERTENSIVE PATIENT

During the day a hypertensive patient may have been taking tranquilizers and other medicines prescribed by his physician. These nerve-quieting drugs are fully as important as any others in controlling hypertension; they relieve strain and promote drowsiness. And in that state the patient is more likely to get into the excellent habit of taking naps. Daily naps are like an elixir to a heart patient, and they will not interfere with sleep at night.

If the hypertensive heart patient is either restless at night or an actual insomniac, then he is a proper candidate for sleeping pills. As I said earlier, he should not hesitate to take them. In fact, he has no choice. The doctor, however brilliant, who neglects to prescribe such medicines is not doing everything he can for his patient.

If your doctor hasn't prescribed sleeping pills, in spite of your complaint that you feel tired from lack of sleep, you had better speak to him about it. If he still insists that he "doesn't believe" in giving his patients sleeping pills, I think it is time to get another medical opinion. Insomnia isn't something that you or your doctor can safely ignore. Look into it, whatever its cause—especially if you are hypertensive.

If you have hypertensive heart disease (or any other disabling condition), your doctor should be a curious cuss. You should trust him less if he is incurious. The doctor who takes the time to talk and ask questions is usually the better doctor. He knows that a good history of the patient's complaints and background is often more important than the physical examination itself. Electrocardiograms, X rays and laboratory tests cannot take the place of a complete history of the patient's illness.

Does the doctor ask you about sex problems? About your relations with your husband (or wife)? About what is really worrying you: finances, children, boredom, fear of disease? About skeletons in your family closet?

The curious doctor knows that he must know the *real* you, for, otherwise, he will be treating you in a maze of buts, ifs, whys and wherefores. Many complaints are based on psychological maladjustments and not on actual physical disease. Psychosomatics is more than a fancy word. Thousands suffer because they keep their "secrets" from their doctor. Then they wonder why he can't or doesn't help.

So it's up to you. Remember that as a hypertensive patient (or as any other sort of patient, for that matter) you haven't really cooperated unless you have stressed the fact that you are tired because you haven't been getting a good night's sleep for weeks and weeks. Unless you tell him, he won't know. And if he doesn't know, he may be way off base in his treatment. And when your doctor's way off base, it's you and not he who is tagged out.

RHEUMATIC HEART DISEASE

The mother of a child with rheumatic fever is worried because she cannot keep him still. "What effect will it have on his heart?" she asks.

There is much we do not know about the complications of rheumatic fever. Why some patients and not others get it in the first place is a mystery. One child gets a strep throat, and it is gone and forgotten; another child has the sore throat, gets over it and then comes down with an attack of rheumatic fever a few weeks later. Why do some children get heart complications during or after their attacks? Why do others escape? Why do some get recurring attacks of rheumatic fever? The truthful answer is that we do not know.

But we do know that antibiotics, if given in full strength and early enough, often prevent serious complications. Every strep throat should be suspect and checked by means of throat cultures. After the first attack of rheumatic fever, penicillin or sulfa drugs taken daily for months and years (or given by injection once monthly) often prevent further attacks and heart damage.

RHEUMATIC FEVER CHILDREN NEED REST

We also know that rheumatic fever patients deserve and need as much rest as they can get. We don't keep them in bed as long as we used to. At times we practically had them chained down for months until their blood counts and sedimentation tests indicated that the infection had completely burned itself out. These days we realize that the unnaturally restricted child wears himself out more by trying to escape from his bed than if we allow him a minimum of exercise.

Nevertheless, the important factor is still rest. Sufficient rest cannot be attained without good, sound sleep night after night. Therefore, as in other forms of heart disease, see that, if necessary, your youngster has sleeping pills.

What I have said about the importance of sleep for cardiac children is as true for adults who have rheumatic heart disease. If you have insomnia, tell your doctor, who will probably prescribe sedatives.

There are many other forms of heart disease: congenital, arteriosclerotic, syphilitic, thyroid, subacute bacterial endocarditis, acute bacterial endocarditis, heart disease as a complication of infections such as pneumonia, etc. But there is not one that isn't greatly counteracted by a good night's sleep. Contrariwise, there isn't one that isn't compounded by insomnia. The heart, like the brain, needs its rest. Complete rest, of course, would be fatal, but a good measure of it—enough to give this faithful worker the periodic relaxation it thrives on—is necessary. And there is no "relaxer" that even approaches sleep in effectiveness.

As always, of course, there are exceptions. For a long time physicians have conjectured that there may be some connection between disturbing dreams and heart attacks such as angina pectoris.

It is readily conceivable that a frightening nightmare might bring on an attack of angina. Thus a recent report from the National Institute of Mental Health reaches the conclusion that "during the R.E.M. period in the early hours of the morning the activity of the autonomic [nervous] system often becomes most intense, inducing what have been called 'autonomic storms,' which may account for the statistically frequent occurrence of heart attacks at this time."

Sleep and heart disease are joined in a common, frustrating mystery that still baffles the scientific investigator. But further research will certainly reveal more of the truth and, as the report of the National Institute of Mental Health makes clear, may make it possible to anticipate and prevent the coronary attacks brought on by nightmares.

10 | Sleep and Chronic Anxiety

DESPITE THESE DAYS of the hydrogen bomb you are probably being facetious if you say that the hyena is the only living thing still capable of laughter. Yet, as you look about you and consider the attitudes of your friends and acquaintances, you know that cheerfulness does not rage through your community in epidemic force.

Anxiety has spread its tentacles remorselessly. All sections of society have felt its tenacious grasp. More than any other ailment (for it is an ailment), anxiety prevents the sufferer from having his rest at night. Anxiety and insomnia are almost synonymous at times. The man or woman who is anxious lies there wide-eyed, the victim of a brain overrun by skittering thoughts and myriads of ideas that whipsaw him from pillar to post.

Jealousy, unrequited love, business worries, resentment, fear of illness, actual disease, family problems, job involvements, ego bruises—one or all can take the measure of sleep.

ANXIOUS PEOPLE ARE THE SAD ONES

Anxious people are usually sad. Like actors', their moods are often cued in by the backdrop and the scenery. Around us are the black curtains of potential war and destruction, so man acts out his part in accordance with the script.

Where are the carefree, spirited days of the twenties? If you are old enough, you recall the easy, casual meetings with people; the bounce and enthusiasm of your friends; the light-heartedness and small talk. There were more parties and more neighborly visiting in those days. And when people got home, they went to bed to sleep and slept. Although insomnia was known to man many years ago, there is little doubt that the problem of sleeplessness has paralleled the increase of anxiety in the world. And since statistics show that there is more insomnia in the United States than elsewhere, we won't be far wrong in guessing that probably we worry more than other peoples.

I am too young to be an old fuddyduddy and too old to be a young hepcat. My vision is somewhere in between. I am open to conviction, but I have my doubts. I wonder if the world is as ebullient, effervescent and optimistic about the future as it was thirty short years ago.

I have sat in at youngsters' parties, and the boys and girls, short- or long-haired, seem more solemn and prematurely grown-up than they were years ago. Solemnity, seriousness and lack of cheer are as catching as measles. The parents of today are overburdened with cares, and the kids inevitably share the mood.

And the universal mood is anxiety about the future.

FEELING SORRY FOR YOURSELF

Man's self-pity is quite disproportionate. Granted that we live in a world experiencing events that presage an all-shattering finale, granted, too, that to live in fear of what may happen is not really to live at all, hopelessness and loss of faith in the future can become ingrained, habit-forms of existence. Man has developed a chronic concern for his tomorrows and has missed the joy of fully living his todays. And what is so important is that, in the process, he misses the joy of a full night's sleep.

Though it may sound grisly—it is a form of shock treatment—I remind those who nurture worry as if it were an inseparable appendage of existence that the worst that can happen to any of us is that we shall die. Come earthquake or no earthquake, nuclear war or no war, the 2½-3 billion of us living today will make place for the several billion of our descendants before a hundred years have passed.

Is that reason enough for living through the present in days of needless dejection and nights spent in trying to sleep?

Man says, "How can I be otherwise in this kind of world?" Having offered this seemingly incontrovertible reason and excuse, he lapses into a mood of spiritless defeat and inner sadness. I contend much of man's dejected apathy is habit—the habit of taking the easy way out. After all, it is hard to be cheerful and optimistic when world events give you an excuse to be otherwise.

It takes less effort to frown than to smile. It is easier to drop the corners of the mouth than to raise them. Look about you on the street, on the buses, in the subway, and make note of the number of placid countenances and smiling faces you see. They are in the minority.

I am not one for wishing that all of us walk about with a perpetual smile on our faces, as if it were imprinted by a rubber stamp. A smile is a pretty thing to behold, but it becomes a tiresome sight when continually lit up; it looks like a pumpkin a week after Halloween.

What I suggest is that we wake up to reality. Time is fleeting. Life is too short to be lived in unnecessary anxiety and sadness. Henry James has shown that although action often follows mood, it is more certain that mood follows action. In other words, you don't run away because you are afraid; rather, you are afraid because you run. Likewise, therefore, you are as often happy because you smile as you smile because you are happy.

HOW ANXIETY AFFECTS SLEEP

How does all this affect your sleep? You fall asleep sooner with a smile on your face than with a frown. Happiness and contentment are the best soporifics.

A workable antidote against mental distress and blackness is to learn how to smile again; to smile outside so that you will feel the cheerfulness within; to develop a philosophy of acceptance of world problems (and your own) so that inner cheerfulness will lie latent even when you are not smiling.

Cheerfulness is positive, not negative. Like playing the piano, it requires unremitting practice and complete control of your feelings. Daily application to this important exercise will have your smile and laughter muscles as supple as the piano player's fingers. If this is cheap five and ten cent philosophy, it works. Try it.

You will note that I haven't said to you, "Stop feeling sorry for yourself." Unfortunately, many insomniacs are trapped by life. Philosophy or no philosophy, they are caught in a mesh of circumstances that, singly or combined, keep them up night after night, trying to figure some way of escape.

MANY CAUSES OF NERVOUSNESS

There are as many causes of nervousness and sleeplessness as there are bundles of nerves. Some of the most desperate cases are the patients who seem trapped by the circumstances of life, with no way of getting out. They seek ways to escape their imminent doom, but everything seems to be closing in on them. Though they ask for help and you are a doctor, you may be helpless to give them succor.

For example, consider the case of the patient who wrote:

> I hope you can give me some advice before I lose my mind. I am very nervous and hardly sleep a wink at night. I'm even afraid to go to sleep because I'm worried. So worried. My face is aging fast with wrinkles around my eyes, although I'm only thirty-five. We have five children (from fifteen years old down to one year). I love them very much. But here's my problem. I don't know what to do for my husband. He's an alcoholic and won't admit it. He becomes befuddled every day on beer and knocks himself out to go to sleep. He is usually out of work and is not a good provider. We're three months overdue on our rent. Gas and light bills are overdue, too. My children are being deprived of their needs. You may notice that I say *my* children. As far as he's concerned, they don't exist.
>
> We fight all the time, and I can't reason with him. We're about to be evicted, but it doesn't bother him. The children are in need of clothes. We live in three sparsely filled rooms. There is hardly a piece of furniture standing. He's now working part-time. He's in debt. He's making our lives miserable. I cannot get help. The county won't help. The employment office got him a job before this one, and he lost it after three days. I am very desperate. Time and again I've told him I'm going to leave him, but he just laughs. He says good riddance. How long must the chil-

dren suffer? He says why should he do anything for his family. I'm not complaining that the children don't have TV. Or that I have a broken-down washing machine someone gave us. All I want is a man in the house to help me raise our children. What I'm really interested in and need desperately is a good night's sleep. How sweet that would be for once. I feel trapped.

What could I say? How could I help? Surely not by giving her a spiel of five cent philosophy and by repeating what I have said about the value of the smile against the frown, etc. She needed specific, practical advice. All I could tell her was that I agreed that she and the children were trapped. But I also told her that the difference between a man and a mouse in a trap is that a man can often find a way out if he does not surrender. I told her she had surrendered. All she was doing was beating her hands against her cell wall and crying out about the indignities being heaped upon her life.

She followed my advice. She joined the organization allied to Alcoholics Anonymous. She went to the secretary of the local medical society, who directed her to willing hands and sympathetic care.

Her husband took strength from her renewed courage and joined Alcoholics Anonymous. He gave up his beer drinking. Apparently insurmountable problems were gradually overcome. He has been on the wagon for the past three years, holding down a job all that time, and the little family is physically and emotionally rehabilitated.

How sweet just one night's sleep would be! This lady is no longer an insomniac because she found ways to overcome her anxieties. She walked out of her trap, with her whole family intact, because she looked for and found a course of action that opened the door for them. If she had continued to rant against her—not imagined—difficulties, her family would still be enmeshed—perhaps completely destroyed. Not all similar problems are soluble, but which is and which isn't are unknown quantities until the effort to escape has been made.

TENSION AND ANXIETY

Tension and anxiety are the handmaidens of insomnia.

Here is a letter from a housewife who says that her main problems are sleeplessness and fear:

> I can't sleep. No wonder: I am full of anxieties. I have more than my share. Here are a few: fear of crowds; fear of having my purse snatched; fear of leaving my house key at home and not locking the door; fear of strangers; fear of riding in airplanes; fear of needles; fear of physicians and dentists, of lightning, of moths, of drowning, of taking a blood test. Is there any way of getting over my insomnia?

Until the tensions, anxieties and phobias are neutralized or actually removed, I fail to see how this patient can possibly expect the relaxation so necessary for a good night's sleep. She says she is afraid of doctors. It seems that her only chance for recovery lies in overcoming this fear. If she is lucky, she will respond to treatment as well as the following patient:

> A miracle has happened to me. I hope you tell this to other readers to give them encouragement. For twenty-

seven years I was housebound by fears. They were so great that if I went more than a few blocks from home, I would lose all sense of orientation. I would get flashing sensations in my eyes and barely see, think I was going blind and fall into a panic.

This fear of mine (I was about twenty-eight when it started) nearly ruined our lives. I spent much money on doctors but received no help. Night after night I stayed awake, wondering if it wouldn't be better to end it all. The doctors told me to "stop worrying," and that my trouble was "only" nerves. Only! Only! I continued in mental agony, and it shadowed the lives of my husband and children. I couldn't engage in their activities or participate in their fun.

Three years ago my son was going to be married, and I didn't know how I could ever make the wedding some distance away. I explained my fears to a new doctor, and he thought I ought to have the benefit of tranquilizers (which, for some reason, my previous doctors refused to prescribe). I took them and went to the wedding. All was well—no panic or loss of orientation.

Since then, taking only two or three a day, I have led a normal life and enjoyed taking trips with my husband. In the past if I had to go someplace, I always backed down at the last minute. Now everything looks wonderful, and I enjoy the scenery. Thank God for an understanding husband and for a doctor who helped me. No one knows what hell on earth is unless he has suffered from fears and has gone night after night without sleep.

(Tranquilizers do not help everyone as they did here; they are not the answer to all nervous problems.)

THE WILL TO FAIL

Some people have only themselves to blame for feeling nervous and sleepless. There is a built-in fault in their mechanism that pulls them in one direction when they know they should be going in another.

Thus, in *Wake Up and Live*—the reading of which, incidentally, I recommend highly as a significant way to increase the mental and physical efficiency of your machine—Dorothea Brande wrote of the *will to fail* as being an inherent part of the makeup of many individuals. Not until they realize the presence of this demoralizing factor in their lives can they possibly improve.

In many instances I have found this to be true. There are people who cannot reach their potential in living because they become exceedingly nervous when they have no apparent reason to feel bad: their ambition pulls them in one direction; the will to fail pulls them in another. They become the center of a maelstrom of emotional imbalance. And you know what that can do to sleep: they become insomniacs.

I have seen housewives who were always tired, nervous and sleepless because they put off their housework until it piled up so high that they were physically and emotionally unable to cope with it—in spite of repeated resolutions not to put it off.

The same cycle has afflicted otherwise capable students, who have failed because the unconscious will to fail made them put off their studying. There was always tomorrow, they thought. Businessmen have come to my office complaining of nervousness, tension and insomnia. Careful inquiry elicited the fact that they, too, were wanting to go in one direction but actually going the opposite way. A sense of proper direction often overcomes nervousness and insomnia more effectively than tranquilizers. Only you can release yourself from the will to fail.

SEXUAL MALADJUSTMENTS

Husbands and wives often lie wide-eyed, unsuspected by the other, because of some sexual maladjustment. In newlyweds and in those who have lived together for many years sexual problems are a common cause of nervousness, unhappiness and insomnia.

Occasionally, I receive letters such as the following from readers of my syndicated newspaper column:

> Dear Dr. Steincrohn:
>
> My wife (nineteen) and I (twenty-eight) have been married for almost nine months and have never yet had sexual intercourse. I love her but think we could love each other even more if we would have better success sexually.
>
> Doctor, my wife told me she did not wish to have intercourse on the first night of our honeymoon, so naturally I was patient and decided to wait. But I am still waiting. Many times when I try to make love to my wife, I get pushed away. Five nights each week I go to bed at 11 P.M., and she stays up until about 1 A.M. so I won't make love to her. The reason I am writing to you is that we are too ashamed to go to anyone else and confess a story like this. We are both becoming nervous wrecks. I am sure neither of us sleeps more than four hours a night. What can we do?

All I could suggest was that it was time they stopped being "too ashamed" to go to anyone. I told them to consult their doctor, which they did. He suggested that they get some books on sexual conduct in marriage. The reading and the frank talks with the family physician gave the wife the answer to the riddle: something even too silly to mention here. In their case insomnia was punctured like a balloon.

A PATIENT GIVES SOME TIPS

It is one thing to sit behind a desk and tell a chronically anxious patient to keep her chin up because "everything will turn out all right in time." It is quite another for a sufferer to give some tips on overcoming chronic anxiety. The following, then, are tips from a patient who has been through the misery these troubled souls encounter day after day and night after night:

> Three years ago I suffered from nervous exhaustion followed by chronic anxiety and inability to sleep well. I found several things that did wonders for me. First of all, realizing that I wasn't alone in the fight—our family doctor was right behind me for support—made all the difference in keeping up my courage.
>
> I started getting lots of rest and taking a nap every afternoon. I began exercising with a TV program. There were times I was so scared I couldn't even get out of a chair. With a little prayer I began to find a little confidence.
>
> I have always hated to cook, but I began to study nutrition to get my mind off myself. It was fun, and I now prepare well balanced meals. This has helped me, too. I used to weigh 194 pounds and am now down to 136. You

see, now that I am less tense, I don't keep nibbling and overeating as I used to do. I discovered that coffee and colas irritated my nerves and cut them out.

To get going in the morning I started taking a shower and rinsing off in cool water; this makes me feel wonderful. I used to take several nerve pills during the day, but I have found that a brisk walk in the evening helps take away the need for so many. I still have a few hills to climb, but I have faith that these can be conquered, too. And other people can conquer them if they keep trying and have faith.

MANY CAUSES FOR ANXIETY

If we could with one sweep of a magic super-duper-tranquilizer pill remove all anxiety from the world, insomnia would receive a terrible blow. But I doubt that it would be a lethal one. I have known people who worried because "things were too good; something bad is bound to happen." So they stayed awake worrying about their good fortune.

Some worry about nothing except loss of sleep. This in itself sets up a block against refreshing sleep. A secretary told me:

Some years ago I used to have quite a time getting to sleep. I would worry about it terribly. At night I would lie in bed trying to go to sleep. I was so worried because I knew that time was going by and I had to get up early in the morning. Sometimes the longer I lay awake, the more tense I would become. What I am getting at is that my problem was caused more by the fear of lack of sleep than by anything else.

My mother was the one who convinced me that there

was nothing to worry about; that my fear was defeating my attempts to fall asleep. She told me that if I wasn't sleepy, not to worry; that if I wasn't sleepy, I didn't need sleep. She told me to lie down, relax, close my eyes and forget about sleep; that such relaxation was practically as good as sleeping. Somehow she convinced me at last.

Seven to eight years have passed since then, and I rarely have any difficulty sleeping. I think this is the trouble with most people who have insomnia. It's the fear of loss of sleep, and nothing else.

Each one of us reacts differently to the same environmental factors. There are football players who are actually fearless when confronted by bone-breaking physical contact yet cringe when they get into an airplane. Sitting next to them may be some little fellow who cringes at the thought of a crushing tackle yet would willingly volunteer to fly to the moon.

FATIGUE CAUSES SLEEPLESSNESS

People who can't sleep are often more tired than they realize. They may be suffering from physiological, psychological or pathological fatigue.

According to Dr. Robert S. Schwab, of Boston, (1) different people can do different things without becoming exhausted, and (2) one person will cope with a set of circumstances in different ways, depending on his energy output and the prevailing conditions. Thus it is not easy to deal with fatigue. It is not merely tiredness. Frequently it is "out of proportion to energy spent; and it will not disappear with rest, sleep or a vacation."

The foremost complaint of people who suffer from

anxiety is fatigue—the almost pathological tiredness that so often prevents sleep. "I was too tired to sleep" is the common cry.

Do you fall asleep burdened by physical exhaustion? Are you overcome by anxiety? Are you full of hate and resentment? Then you are bound to awake irritable and filled with inescapable fatigue.

FIND THE REASON FOR FATIGUE

Taking pills for your insomnia may be as ineffectual as pouring water on a gasoline blaze. Your job is to ferret out the basic reasons for your anxiety. It's not easy, but like any other important project, it deserves a good try. Otherwise, you may live out your life as an insomniac.

Have your doctor make certain that your fatigue and sleeplessness are not due to actual organic disease, for tiredness is often the first symptom of unsuspected illness. We find it in patients who have heart disease, tuberculosis, diabetes, hypothyroidism and other conditions.

It is important to eliminate the cause, whatever it is. I recall a prominent businessman who came in complaining of what he called "deathly fatigue," which caused his insomnia. On digging down into his history, we discovered that he was unaware that he became tired at the very sight of his partner, with whom he was closeted all day, every day, at his office.

His insomnia disappeared when he sold out to his partner. "That's the best sale I ever made in my life," he said.

Unfortunately, insomnia caused by hate and resentment is not always so easily neutralized.

11 | Sleep and Ulcer Trouble

WE DO NOT KNOW what causes a stomach ulcer, but we surely know what makes it worse. It feeds on resentment. And resentment never walks on longer legs than when it stalks through a mind filled with flitting thoughts during the long nights of insomnia. The long dark hours breed and nourish resentment.

For years I treated a vice-president of a large corporation for duodenal ulcer. And since the treatment was unsuccessful, the decision for or against operation loomed, for he had already had one severe hemorrhage, which required a raid on the blood bank to save him, and his pain was severe and unrelenting, except when he took food and medications to combat his hyperacidity. Yet he argued:

> I'm too afraid of the knife. I won't consent to operation. I won't let you take away a part of my stomach. I'd rather die off the operating table than on it. Call me a coward or whatever you will, but don't blame me. I have friends who wouldn't get into an elevator for a million dollars. You can't blame them for having claustrophobia. And you can't blame me for being so scared of the knife. Even when my wife picks one up to carve food, I feel a sweat coming on. It's a phobia.

I told him I sympathized. We'd try for a while longer to keep on with medical management. He consented to give up cigarettes and alcohol, to watch his diet more carefully, to take more frequent vacations and to let down on his work at the office.

But I had a vague feeling that something was missing, that he wasn't really confiding in me or telling me everything that was on his mind. I had the impression that something had been nagging at him for a long while, and that he was keeping it to himself.

"You have been a most cooperative patient," I said. "Except for one thing: you haven't come clean. You haven't told me just how you feel about your family, your friends, your work, your business associates. It's important for me to know these things. I must know why you are not improving. A person's psychological makeup often interferes with his good health. What is eating you that you haven't told me about?"

I recall that consultation very well. He sat still and his face became white; he didn't say anything for a minute. I sat waiting, knowing that he would soon begin to tell.

He talked about his wife and three children with great affection (I knew they were a happy family). He had many friends, he said, and was apparently a well-regarded citizen in his community. Then he began to talk faster. It was imperceptible at first, but soon the words began to spill out one after the other, like scared rabbits scattered by sudden gunfire. The gist of what he admitted follows:

> So you see I have everything to live for. I'm only in my forties, happy family, many friends, and a good job. . . . I wonder if my job can have anything to do with my ulcer. It's a good job, but for the past two years I have been very unhappy in it. I know why, although I've never

even mentioned it to a soul until now—not even to my wife. In fact, everyone thinks I've been a great sport about it.

I'm referring to the fact that I was in line for promotion to the presidency of our organization two years ago. Everyone was congratulating me prematurely. At the annual meeting they announced that the new president was to be a friend of mine who had only been with the firm for a few years and had a job way down on the scale compared with mine.

I've actually hated that guy since then. Now that I think of it, it wasn't long after that I began to have my stomach pains. I resented him more than I thought it was possible for one human being to hate another. Although I knew he was innocent, that he was greatly surprised when he got the post, he became my target. To this day he doesn't know that whenever I meet him and show him a full set of teeth in a wide smile, I'm hating his guts. All the while people have been congratulating me on being a good loser. Even my wife marvels at my saintly magnanimity. She can't get over how well I've taken it. But I wonder, now that you've mentioned the psychological aspects of ulcer, if this resentment of mine hasn't played a part in it.

Do you know, doctor, it has gotten so bad that I can't sleep at night? I lie there, thinking of the poor guy and hating him with relish. Is it any wonder I have to get up about three o'clock every morning to take some milk to put out the fire in my stomach?

There you have it first hand: a confession good, not only for his soul, but also for his stubborn ulcer. From that moment he began to improve. Although ten years later he met the knife when he underwent an urgent operation to remove a badly inflamed appendix (which operation he accepted without undue pressure), he has never had to undergo surgery for his ulcer. Clinical and X-ray evidence give proof that it has healed.

The cure was simple. At least the plan was. He was told not to hold any resentment against the new boss anymore. It wasn't easy at first. But he became an apt pupil. I think he first saw good reason for giving it a try when I told him about the experiments conducted at Cornell a number of years ago.

EXPERIMENT AT CORNELL

The subject of the experiment was a man who had a permanent hole in his stomach from an accident he sustained as a boy. This man worked in the medical laboratory at Cornell, and he was also paid to be a sort of guinea pig for psychological experiments. Thus one day the scientists accused him of destroying the results of an important laboratory experiment and put him on the table to observe the inside wall of his stomach through the hole as he became angry at what was a false accusation.

Since he was innocent, he resented the accusation. And the researchers saw that the sudden resentment caused the mucous membranes of his stomach wall to turn red and angry. Areas of pinpoint hemorrhages in the stomach formed under the investigators' eyes. Here was scientific evidence of what resentment can do to a stomach—and to many other organs in the body.

The scientists then told the man that they had only been

fooling. They had been using him, they said, to determine what anger and resentment can do to a human stomach. At this he relaxed immediately, laughing at the "joke," and within minutes his stomach had returned to normal.

As I told our vice-president with the ulcer of this experiment, his eyes widened in disbelief. "Can it be possible?" he said. Not only possible but likely, I told him. Just think, I said, what resentment has done to your stomach. Your resentment hasn't been a fleeting thing. Day after day and, what's worse, night after night you have actually been eating up the walls of your own stomach. Call it a form of cannibalism. Unremittingly, unceasingly, you have been feeding your own innards to the wolves of hate.

I told him the best way to get over it was by taking the brave step, by walking directly up to the problem and facing it unflinchingly. Then he would improve. And he did.

He invited his "friend," the boss, to his home and told him everything. He confessed his hatreds, his long period of resentment and his apparent happiness in his job. The two became closer friends than they had ever been. Our man's ulcer improved long before the boss appointed him executive vice-president. When resentment went out of the window, sweet nature took over.

Medically speaking, one of the most important phases of the cure was establishing normal sleep patterns in the patient. Although he had resolved no longer consciously to resent his friend, he found it difficult to keep his resolve at night.

"When you lie in bed, unable to sleep, it's easier said than done to keep bad thoughts from flitting all over the place," he said. "It's dark, everyone else is asleep, it's quiet and you lie there fighting insomnia, waiting for daylight to break so you will stop thinking bad thoughts."

In his case, sleeping pills were the most useful medication for his duodenal ulcer. All he needed was one Seconal capsule every night for about three weeks. He stopped taking them without difficulty and has never used sleeping pills since. He did the same with the tranquilizer I prescribed for a few months. All he takes now for sleep is some warm milk. His theory is that the warm milk gives him a good night's sleep because it must unconsciously bring back to him the pleasures and security of babyhood, when warm milk and good sleep were so closely associated in the mind of the infant.

The vice-president's case is but one of hundreds. Too many sufferers from ulcers feed their ulcers on resentment while feeding their stomachs on ineffectual offerings of milk and cream.

If you have an ulcer, do not be a "coverup man." Tell the doctor your innermost animosities. That's what he's for. Family doctors and psychiatrists should be repositories of the innermost secrets, fears and problems of patients who are repressing their resentments. The patient who tells his doctor all helps the doctor cure his insomnia and ulcer at the same time.

12 | Sleep and Thyroid Disorders

LAZY THYROID

HE SLEEPS MOST OF THE DAY; he can hardly keep his eyes open. But he stays up most of the night. I call it sleeping "backwards." And I am not talking about a young infant. It's my twenty-two-year-old son, who can't seem to get enough sleep during the day and is wide-awake at night.

He is a senior at college. How he has been able to pass beats me. He can't even stay awake during lectures. His professors overlook his sleeping only because he hands in brilliant examination papers. (He takes a half-dozen cups of coffee and several Benzedrine tablets to stay awake during exams.)

He is always very tired for lack of sleep at night. He drags himself down to breakfast, half asleep. When he comes home at about 3 P.M., he still seems to be sleepy and could, if he had time, go back to bed and sleep the rest of the afternoon. I've seen him sleep eighteen hours at a stretch after he has been up night after night for weeks. He seemed to lack energy all through high school, too.

Is there anything we can do? He hasn't been to a doctor for years because he seems so healthy otherwise.

I told her that the two most important things to check on were the thyroid and the possibility that he was suffering from narcolepsy. In his case, further study put the finger on a lazy thyroid: it was not putting out sufficient thyroid hormone. When her son had taken three grains of thyroid hormone every day for a few months, his sleep habits were reversed: he slept at night and stayed awake during the day.

Often I have heard people say, "All the doctor keeps saying is that there is nothing wrong, and that my condition is due to nerves. Do you wonder that I dislike seeing him? I sometimes wish he could find something like an ulcer or even worse, so my family won't keep thinking I'm just another chronic complainer."

In this light, consider this letter:

> Some time ago you mentioned a letter from a woman who was so tired that she found herself hating her family sometimes, although she put her whole life into serving them. I wish you would write on the necessity of helping those in the family who constantly complain of being tired. I know just how that woman felt.
>
> Much as I have loved my own family, many times my tears would fall into the dishwater because although I was so exhausted, my constant complaints of weariness were ignored by those who, though they really loved me, serenely played games while I worked on far past my strength, year after year.
>
> Finally, I was utterly shocked by my daughter, who loved me devotedly, when she said, "When you complain of being tired, we never pay any attention, because you've been tired as long as we can remember, but Daddy has been so well and strong that when he says he's tired, it scares us to death."
>
> At last, after all these suffering years, a doctor has

found a cause for my chronic fatigue and insomnia. I have hypothyroidism. The basal metabolism test didn't pick it up, but a test they call the protein-bound iodine test showed what was the trouble with me.

I now take thyroid extract every day, and although I still get tired once in a while, what a difference! My children and husband flutter around me as if they were mother hens and I the chick. It's a wonderful feeling to have proper sympathy from your loved ones. And how gratifying to go to bed and find some good sleep rather than having to face night after night of battling with that old devil insomnia.

HYPOTHYROIDISM OFTEN OVERLOOKED

I have seen scores of patients with undiagnosed hypothyroidism. It is often overlooked because all cases do not have the typical textbook symptoms. In the easily recognized case of underactive gland the patient complains of fatigue. But in addition there is increased sensitivity to cold. The patients can't stand the slightest drop in temperature. Their skin is coarse. Their hair is dry and falling out. The pulse is slow. The cholesterol in their blood is often higher than normal. They slow up mentally. Sometimes there is puffiness of the eyelids. They react slowly and live much below the level of their normal potential.

I have also noted that hypothyroid patients may have a reversal of sleep habits. They are sleepy during the day and wakeful at night. This may be owing to the fact that they sleep themselves out during the day and therefore do not sleep at night. But perhaps there's a glandular reason. In any case, given treatment with proper dosage of thyroid extract, they develop and fulfill their energy potentials during the day and sleep at night.

I advise every person who suffers from fatigue, especially if it is complicated by insomnia, to have a complete study of his thyroid gland. There are many reasons for tiredness other than thyroid gland underactivity, but it should not be allowed to go unrecognized as often as it is.

Sometimes the hypothyroidism becomes so marked that the patient becomes almost incapacitated. One patient was admitted to a mental institution because doctors were certain that she had a psychosis. On studying her after her entry, however, they found she had myxedema. Proper thyroid administration transformed her from a mental patient into a normal human being in three to four months. One of her outstanding symptoms had been insomnia. After treatment this disappeared.

The cases that fool us are the marginal or subliminal ones. The patient does not exhibit the usual features of hypothyroidism. All he says is that he can't sleep and that he is tired. He takes tonics, vitamins and dozens of other medications on his own. Thus, not until the insomniac submits himself for medical survey is it likely that the discovery of a lazy thyroid will be made.

OVERACTIVE THYROID GLAND

Hyperthyroidism, overactive thyroid gland, is also a cause of insomnia. People suffering from hyperthyroidism are *driven*. They can't seem to relax. The pulse is rapid and often irregular. The skin is moist and warm. They may have palpitation and heart skips. Their muscles tire easily. Sometimes they complain of spells of diarrhea. Their eyes are wide open and starey. They cannot sit still. They fidget.

They have a finger tremor, so slight that you have to examine carefully to see it. Loss of weight, despite an excellent appetite, and sleeplessness round out the typical picture.

Often, however, the symptoms are not typical. It is not easy to make the diagnosis unless one always bears in mind that malfunction of the thyroid gland is masking itself as something else.

For example, here is a patient who complained of symptoms apparently unrelated to hyperthyroidism:

> I am fifty-eight years old and have complained of insomnia intermittently for the past two years. I have been in excellent health except that I've been more nervous than usual. I fall asleep quite easily, but my wife tells me I sleep restlessly. After three to four hours of fitful sleep I wake up and often lie there until it is almost time to get up. It is a vicious circle because the next night I am extremely tired, fall asleep earlier than usual and then wake again after a few hours. My doctor prescribed sleeping tablets, but I don't take them regularly.
>
> Sometimes I get up to drink a glass of milk; sometimes I can read myself back to sleep; sometimes the radio helps if there is a program of soft, instrumental music. Although I smoke freely during the day, I do not smoke at night.
>
> My insomnia doesn't seem to be affected by the type of bed or bedding or by the temperature of the room, unless it is extremely hot or cold. In my neighborhood there is a good deal of street noise, but this does not seem to rouse me. However, the slightest noise within the apartment, even the scratching of a mouse, will have me wide-awake immediately—heart pounding.
>
> I used not to be a worrier, but over the past few years

I have changed. The least little thing will make me afraid and set my heart beating fast. In fact, it beats fast all the time, even when I go to bed in a normal state of cheerfulness. I become panicked when I wake up in the early morning hours. Everything unpleasant that has ever happened or that might happen to me or to those dear to me comes to plague me at these times and prevents a return to normal sleep. That's when I reach for a soporific book, the dullest I can find.

What or whether I eat or drink before bedtime seems to make little difference. I may sleep soundly after three cups of coffee, or waken and toss about after a pint of hot milk or a beer. Incidentally, I can't understand why I have lost over twenty pounds, because my appetite is voracious. I have become distinctly thinner, in spite of all my efforts to reverse the trend.

I said that this patient's symptoms were apparently unrelated to hyperthyroidism. Insomnia was the standout. Yet, he had some of the cardinal symptoms: loss of weight, good appetite, nervousness, rapid pulse and inability to relax.

A high protein-bound iodine test and a basal metabolic rate of over thirty-five established the diagnosis of hyperthyroidism. After due preparation he had a thyroidectomy. Gradually he began to gain weight; he lost his nervousness, his heart-pounding stopped; and he no longer suffered from insomnia.

Never forget the thyroid: it may be underactive or overactive, and either condition may cause insomnia.

13 | Sleep and Allergies

WAITING IN THE LOBBY of a theater before a matinee performance, I heart the loud whine of sirens. An ambulance braked at the entrance, and two men hurried into the theater with a stretcher. Within minutes they were on their way out. On the stretcher a woman received an injection as they carried her toward the ambulance.

I talked later to a doctor who had been a member of the audience. "I don't know how it happened," he said. "But a bee got in there somehow and stung this woman. Within a minute or two she was gasping for air. If I hadn't had some adrenaline handy, she might have died before we got her to a hospital. In fact, if the adrenaline hadn't worked, I wouldn't have hesitated to do a tracheostomy right on the spot."

This is a story of allergy and of how it can sometimes cause an acute emergency. But it's an old story. Somehow people have gotten the idea that it is something new in medicine. But allergy goes way back in history. There's evidence in hieroglyphics on Egyptian tablets that a King Menes died of the sting of a hornet a few thousand years before the birth of Christ.

Even Hippocrates knew of asthma and often said that patients who had headaches should not be given milk. He may not have known the actual mechanism of allergy, with its allergens (irritating substances) and its antibodies (the body's protective substances), but he must have been aware that in some persons the body resents the entrance of certain irritants.

We know now that these allergens may enter the body through the nose or mouth by breathing; through the skin; through the stomach and intestines; or by secondary infection.

Thus hay fever and asthma may result from breathing the pollen of giant ragweed. If you are sensitive to some substance where you work, you may develop contact dermatitis. If you are sensitive to chicken, you may get a severe headache, nausea or vomiting. If you develop sensitivity to bacteria that once infected you, you may later develop an allergy to them. In fact, one theory about the cause of rheumatic fever is that the body becomes sensitized to streptococci and a few weeks later develops joint swelling and the other symptoms of rheumatic fever.

Any one of the types of allergy I have mentioned may interfere with sleep.

HAY FEVER INTERFERES WITH SLEEP

At the height of his attack, the patient with hay fever will tell you he wishes he had an ulcer or something worse rather than his own discomforts. The hay fever sufferer was looked upon years ago as some sort of clown. His reddened nose, the sniffles and sneezes, the mounds of tissue discarded, the complaints unheard and minimized—all contributed to the "funny" picture of hay fever. Not until it became more widespread, affecting millions, did the scoffers (many of whom turned out to be hay fever victims themselves) appreciate the trials of the allergy patient.

Like many other patients, the hay fever patient suffers

most intensely at night. During the day the physical butt of outlandish symptoms that try his patience, he crawls into bed at night with a prayer that he may have some surcease. He is probably already filled up with antihistamine tablets that have dulled his thinking and caused him to fight off sleep while still at work and with aches and pains as if he had the flu. The mucous membranes inside his nose are turgid and swollen and close off the normal nasal air intake. He must breathe through his open mouth.

This unsatisfactory method of securing his oxygen supply causes his mouth to become dry and uncomfortable. He continues to sneeze and discard mounds of tissue napkins. He curses the luck that has singled him out as a hay fever victim.

He may throw back his head and spill a few drops of medicine into his nostrils or blow in some antihistamine and adrenaline with an atomizer. Often he will use Benzedrine or one of its counterparts to find relief. The latter may dry up secretions and open air passages temporarily, but it has a way of keeping the patient awake most of the night.

I tell hay fever patients to respect this pesky illness. Rather than go to the drug store and experiment with a few antihistamines, cough mixtures or nose drops, I advise them to stop guessing and self-treatment and to let a doctor determine the real cause of their trouble. In stubborn cases only an allergist can hope to overcome the distress.

DIAGNOSIS IS IMPORTANT

Diagnosis is important. What is the cause? Is it giant ragweed? Mango? Mold or mildew? Is it your own perfume, face powder or shaving cream?

Unless he determines the cause, your doctor is as helpless as you are to overcome or even neutralize hay fever. He determines what the culprit is by various means. You have heard of the scratch tests and patch tests which he uses to discover your sensitivities, but he also uses special blood tests and insists on your giving him a complete history of yourself.

Suppose the cause is dust. Admittedly, you cannot live in this world without being exposed to it, but your job is to eradicate as much of it as possible from your home. Your bedroom, especially, should be dust free. The doctor, like a detective, will run down every possible source of it: walls, floor, ceiling, books, windows, molding, furniture, shoes, magazines, clothes and scores of other sources.

In addition to desensitizing you with increasingly strong injections of dust antigens, he will concentrate on ridding your bedroom of allergenic dust and mold. There is where you win or lose your nightly battle with insomnia.

If you have severe hay fever or asthma owing primarily to dust sensitivity, here are some practical suggestions that will help. Your own doctor will make the specific changes necessary in your sleeping environment, and only the trained allergist can tell you what to do about it all.

NEUTRALIZING DUST ALLERGY

Never stay in a room that is being cleaned. Many a severe attack of hay fever or asthma has been precipitated by sitting there reading while dust mops and vacuum cleaners kick up a storm. And stay out of the recently cleaned room. Air it well first by opening all windows wide. Air conditioning is the answer for some patients. However, many others simply cannot feel comfortable with it.

Preferably, sleep alone. One bed in the room is ideal during (and to prevent) attacks. Remove all dust collectors: curtains, carpets and extra furnishings. Clean the walls and ceiling, even scrub the bed-springs. Have someone scrub the floors and woodwork and do a weekly job on closets and their innards. It is a good idea to keep the bedroom door closed; do not invite an invasion of dust from the rest of the house. Throw out all stuffed furniture and, of course, remove all carpeting. Cover your matresses and pillows with allergen-proof materials. Use washable bedspreads and blankets.

Don't go rummaging in attics or storerooms. Even a few minutes of such exposure to excessive dust has brought on severe attacks.

Feather and kapok are common irritants to allergic persons. If you can't eliminate them entirely, then at least try to render them dustproof. Do a complete inventory of your quilts, cushions, mattresses, pillows, bedding. Horse dander is another cause of severe reactions in sensitive people who use mattresses, pillows or blankets made of horse hair. Removal will often result in amazing improvement.

ALL KINDS OF ALLERGIES

Camel hair coats and goat hair blankets or rugs are frequent causes of allergic attacks. Nevertheless, it is easier to get rid of these than it is to part with a pet parakeet when you are sensitive to bird feathers or to say good-bye to a family pet because your doctor has discovered that you are allergic to dog or cat hair.

A lot of trouble, isn't it, to try to get a night's sleep? Nevertheless, unless you overcome or neutralize the allergy, you will be sleepless night after night. Besides, your hay fever may progress into asthma, and your asthma may become an even more serious problem.

As I mentioned, an allergic reaction may involve your skin and cause severe dermatitis. This reaction, too, will keep you up, because of the intense itching. In the same way, a food allergy may give you migraine and prevent sleep or produce nausea or vomiting and keep you up half the night.

Remember that allergy, that all-inclusive word that covers so much misery, is another of insomnia's allies. Tranquilizers, sleeping pills, sedatives, antihistamines may help temporarily. But the lasting relief that allows sleep comes only with proper diagnosis and treatment for the allergy. It is not easy to discover the allergen, but it is worth trying to find it, for it is important that you do your best to prevent such complications as chronic bronchitis, asthma or emphysema—a stubborn, tenacious trio of lung invaders that deprive millions of us from getting a good night's sleep.

14 | Sleep and the Menopause

ANOTHER NOT UNCOMMON COMPLAINT is loss of sleep during the change of life. Whether it be in a woman's well-accepted menopause or in a man's still debated "male climacteric," loss of sleep is a prominent complaint. The nervousness and depression that sometimes accompany these changes aggravate insomnia, and vice versa.

Therefore, as important as hormones are the tranquilizers and sedatives the patient needs to get a fairly sizable quota of sleep and relaxation at night. But it is important to make the correct diagnosis: before we treat a man for the male climacteric, we must be sure that no other organic condition is simulating it.

I recall one man in his mid-fifties who was referred to me because his associates found him a burden in their business. Formerly dependable and astute, he had become disoriented: his memory went back on him and he lost his reasoning power. Organically, he seemed sound. There was no trouble in his heart, blood pressure or kidneys. But he was undoubtedly a sick man. What was it?

I thought he was going through the male climacteric, and hoped to help him with hormones, energizers, tranquilizers or electroshock therapy. But that was not the trouble. He had cerebral atherosclerosis. He was developing senile changes because of the disturbed blood supply in his brain. Unfortunately nothing seemed to help, and he went steadily downhill and died of a complicating pneumonia.

The diagnostic finger does, however, sometimes point correctly at the male change. Within a few months a handsome, alert, gracious and charming man becomes untidy, irritable and forgetful. You rule out every other possible cause you can think of. Nothing else shows up. So you prescribe male hormones, tranquilizers and energizers. If these do not help, you use electroshock therapy. Usually the man is reconverted into a more nearly normal human being.

In these cases the first evidence of beginning recovery is usually this statement from the family or patient: "Sleeping much better." Unless these patients obtain their sleep, it is doubtful that they will recover. So the doctor must not hesitate to prescribe strong soporifics, and the patients must not hesitate to take them.

A doctor's job is both to heal and to save life and to bring comfort wherever and whenever he can. In most cases, prescribing sex hormones and tranquilizers will convert the most uncomfortable woman into a placid, happy person. (As it often does for the patient in premenstrual tension, too.) I often wish that doctors who are therapeutic nihilists could suffer the distress and irritations some of their patients endure, and especially that they would have to go to their office and make their hospital rounds after nights of insufficient sleep. Then they might change their minds about withholding medication and "letting nature take its course."

Too many physicians minimize chronic loss of sleep as being of little consequence. But insomnia can gradually add up to a mountain of trouble.

Unfortunately, not all women can safely take hormones because of the presence of specific contra-indications. But most can. And they deserve the relief hormones bring in comfort and restfulness, and good sleep promises them that.

15 | Sleep and Mental Disorders

IT IS VERY COMMON for people to feel uncomfortable and yet not to know, or accept, the cause of the trouble. It is, therefore, not unusual for such unhappy people to get on the medical merry-go-round, visiting countless doctors, hoping for some satisfactory explanation of their miseries.

For example, consider this letter:

Dear Dr. Steincrohn:

I am thirty-eight years old. My chief complaint is inability to sleep through the night. I keep waking up and find it difficult to fall asleep again. At times I feel faint, and my heart seems to give a couple of hard thuds and then it will beat fast for a half hour. You can understand that this isn't conducive to good sleep, either.

I have been to many doctors. All they do is give me a bottle of nerve medicine and say it's "just nerves." I asked for an electrocardiogram, blood sugar tests and X rays. All are normal. But I am very annoyed with doctors who say nothing but "it's just your nerves!"

In reply, I agreed that nothing irritates and depresses a patient more than this sort of statement from a doctor. The patient leaves the doctor's office not knowing where or to whom to turn next. He still suffers. All the satisfaction he can get is to know that he isn't really organically sick.

But what is the doctor to say? He cannot manufacture illness that isn't there. In any case, when a patient has harmless heart skips and vague aches in the chest, the doctor is happy to be able to say, "There's nothing organically wrong with your heart."

But he must not stop there. In addition to prescribing sedatives, tranquilizers and other medicines, it is the doctor's responsibility to try to ferret out the real cause of the patient's anxieties and to treat him for them. Sometimes he can do it all by himself; in severe cases of insomnia and nervousness he may need the help of a psychiatrist.

The doctor should be as sympathetic to the organically sound, nervous patient as he is to the patient who "really" has organic trouble. Remember, insomnia is no respecter of persons: it attacks the sick and the apparently healthy who suffer from nerves.

NERVOUS ANXIETY

Anxiety is a potent factor in upsetting sleep. Whether the anxiety is brought about by actual organic illness or by "just nerves" is unimportant; what *is* important is that the insomnia not be treated as something unimportant. With this in mind consider the following letter:

> How is a person to know whether he merely has "bad" nerves or whether there is something actually wrong with him? For years I was told I had a "nervous stomach." Then I finally had two jim-dandy attacks that alerted my doctor to the possibility it might be something else. It was gall bladder disease. But after the operation I began to have eating problems: more tranquilizers and a diagnosis of "nerves" again.

Then one day I casually mentioned to my doctor that I had dark stools. Tests showed that I had ulcers (two of them, duodenal and gastric). I now stick to my diet and feel fine, except for sleeplessness and exhaustion. I'm tired all the time. That is not surprising when you consider that I never sleep undisturbed through a night. I'm up at least a half-dozen times, and I have a half-dozen separate fights to fall asleep again.

I'm tired of it and of myself. I want to start feeling good and living again, and I can't without a good night's sleep. Incidentally, I love life. I'm happiest when I'm busy, and I enjoy people. I am active in church and P.T.A. activities and take an active part in pet local issues. I also attend courses at high school at night. I don't want, you see, to live the life of an invalid.

I have enthusiasm enough for two people, and, thank God, I've never lost my sense of humor. But I hate to think of what I'm doing to my nice family (husband and three children) by being exhausted and sleepless all the time.

Incidentally, I eat nutritionally sound meals, do not smoke or drink, take three cups of coffee a day, get plenty of rest (except at night) and have hobbies. But I still sound like an old woman, and I'm only thirty-seven. Therein lies my tale of woe. I know it's not the worst story you've ever heard, but it's *my* worst story. What now? How about some sleep?

To this woman I replied, in effect: many patients, like yourself, being treated for "nervous stomach" have some organic trouble. For that reason many doctors leave the "nerves" diagnosis till last. Only after they have made a comprehensive effort to make certain that gall bladder disease is not present, that there is no ulcer, no hiatal hernia, no intestinal trouble, no liver or pancreas trouble, no sign of any one of a score of conditions that might cause "stomach trouble" will they diagnose "nerves."

But this is not as easy as it sounds. Sometimes organic disease evades us. For example, gall bladder or ulcer trouble may "hide" on X rays. The findings may not be definite, or they may be too obscure for a definite diagnosis. That is why repeat X rays are so often necessary.

Moreover, it is possible, as your case history shows, to have a combination of organic disease and functional illness. Consider the progress of your own case.

Both your gall bladder and your ulcers have been treated successfully, yet you complain of the original symptoms of "nervous stomach." This indicates that you have an overlay of anxiety producing the very symptoms of exhaustion, nervousness and insomnia that still trouble you.

My advice? It's just a guess, but I think you are attempting to crowd too much into twenty-four hours. You are one of those energetic persons who try to live thirty hours in twenty-four. Your appetite for doing things is much greater than your body's capacity to do them.

Some of us must resign ourselves to the fact that we came off the assembly line a bit below par in energy reserves; we must learn to live within the limits of what we can do without getting exhausted. I think that it is most important that you cut down the nonessentials (although you enjoy them) in order to conserve your energy. Become an energy-miser. Otherwise you will go through life unable to enjoy the simple things that bring us so much comfort and satisfaction, for example, a good night's rest.

DOCTORS SHOULD NOT MINIMIZE IMPORTANCE OF INSOMNIA

In *The Horse and Buggy Doctor*, Arthur E. Hertzler, M.D., writes: "Nothing in all the range of human complaints excites my sympathy so much as sleeplessness. The eternal night. He who conquers this for his patient, more than in any other situation, has contributed to the alleviation of human suffering."

Doctors, as well as patients, are now beginning to recognize the importance of sleep for the well and the sick. In fact, Russian scientists have been conducting experiments on dogs to prove that prolonged sleep causes rejuvenation. One dog, in which they induced sleep for approximately three months, even regained its productive ability and outlived by a half-dozen years other dogs of the identical breed.

The Russians have been using a similar technique on humans to restore their vigor and well-being, especially in neurotic patients who suffer from depression. The treatment involves using sleeping pills to keep the patients asleep from twelve to twenty-four hours daily for a period of three weeks.

Dr. Wilfred Dorfman, editor-in-chief of *Psychosomatics*, has noted: "In neurotic depression, there is often difficulty in getting to sleep; in endogenous [involutional or manic depressive] depression, the patient may experience some difficulty in falling asleep, but the really distressing aspect of this insomnia is early awakening after which the patient finds it impossible to get to sleep again."

But scientists work on the assumption that nothing is impossible. And, in addition to the Russians, many researchers are experimenting with producing a minor degree of hibernation.

EXPERIMENTS IN PROLONGED SLEEP THERAPY

Some insight into the methods and results of prolonged sleep therapy is given by H. Azima, M.D., of McGill University, Montreal:

> Prolonged sleep treatment appears to be most useful for management of manic states, agitated depression, acute schizophrenia, agitated paranoid states, mixed psychoneuroses, and anxiety hysterias. Chlorpromazine or promazine medication should be tried for patients in psychotic states before sleep treatment is instituted. . . . Sleep lasting 20-22 hours per day is induced with a combination of barbiturates and chlorpromazine. The basic formula consists of 100 mg. of Nembutal, 150 mg. of Amytal Sodium or Veronal, and 50 mg. of chlorpromazine or 100 mg. of promazine. Patients are aroused three times daily, and the amount of medication is adjusted according to the degree of wakefulness, which is measured by response to light and sound and ability to talk, move and eat. The dosage required and the smoothness of sleep depend mainly upon the willingness of the patient to accept the treatment. Duration of the treatment is preferably fifteen to twenty days. . . .
>
> Nursing care: during the waking period, temperature, pulse, blood pressure, and respiration are recorded. Then the patient is moved out of bed, washed, and fed. At least 1500 calories and 2,000 cc. of fluid should be taken daily; fluid intake is adjusted according to output. Vitamins are given parenterally. A half hour before meals five units of insulin is administered to increase appetite. Milk of magnesia is given every other day, and colonic irrigation is performed if elimination does not occur in two days; if the patient does not urinate, catheterization is performed as necessary. Between waking periods the position of the patient is changed every two hours. Oxygen-carbon

dioxide mixtures are given if the patient's breathing becomes shallow.

Results of sleep treatment: of 23 schizophrenics 4 showed great and 12 moderate improvement. Of 14 manic depressive patients 6 showed great and 4 moderate improvement. Of 29 neurotics, 6 were greatly and 5 moderately improved.*

From this it is clear that the results of prolonged sleep therapy, although often quite efficacious, are by no means infallible. So many people are neurotic, or even psychotic, that if this treatment were to work for all patients with neuroses, millions would sleep away their phobias and hallucinations. Perhaps if Attila, Hitler, Mussolini and scores of similar madmen had been "put under" for a few weeks of continuous sleep therapy, the world might have been spared their depredations. If we could transform such people into human hedgehogs and put them out of circulation for a few months each year, their waking hours might be more mellow and less given to thoughts of mass murder.

Although the hedgehog hibernates for about seven months a year, he never seems to get enough sleep. Even during the five summer months he sleeps about eighteen hours a day. He is really only active about two months a year; the other ten months he spends in hibernation and sleep. (I wonder about his thyroid function or tendency to narcolepsy!)

LACK OF SLEEP MAY BE SERIOUS

I have observed numerous patients in whom lack of sleep was the forerunner and a part of severe mental illness. When I delved into their histories, inability to get a good night's sleep was their foremost complaint. I recall some who refused to take sedatives or sleeping pills. Their depression

* *Diseases of the Nervous System*, 1958.

became so deep that they attempted suicide, sometimes successfully. Many such cases, I believe, might have found an antidote against destruction in sleep.

Sleeping pills, therefore, should not be considered only as treatment drugs; they are prevention drugs, too. As sleep is the healer, so it is the preventer. Mental patients may be helped by sleeping pills, but, even more important, people are prevented from becoming mental patients by the early and wise use of hypnotics and sedatives.

It bears repeating, therefore, that people should not be afraid to take "dope" under the care of their physician. Many persons think that the medicine itself may harm the organs. For example:

> Dear Dr. Steincrohn:
>
> A number of months ago you wrote about the use of chlorpromazine in the management of elderly people who have become mental problems. I asked you about my father, who is in his seventies and has become irritable, hard to please, sleepless and far from neat in his habits. You said, why not take up the question of using this medicine with your doctor. I did, and he said it wouldn't hurt to try. I write to report a miraculous metamorphosis. My father is now gentle, sweet and almost his former self of twenty years ago. There's only one question in my mind. Is such a powerful medicine liable to cause damage to the system? I've heard that it may affect the liver.

It is true that chlorpromazine sometimes produces undesired reactions in the blood, liver and nervous system. But so do many other valuable drugs. The remarkable and encouraging thing is that these reactions occur relatively infrequently. Take this seventy-year-old man, for instance. The letter indicates that he has been taking the drug for a few months. If he has not had jaundice (which may indicate hepatitis) in that period, chances are that he will not have this trouble later. When a reaction does occur, it usually does so during the first two months of treatment. In any case, his doctor has probably taken an occasional blood test to check on any reactions. All in all, the writer may be thankful for this helpful drug that has given her father sleep and comfort.

In my experience, chlorpromazine has helped people of all age groups. Chlorpromazine treatment often calms unmanageable children and middle-aged neurotics, and psychotics frequently become so tractable under chlorpromazine that they are discharged from institutions long before expected and are able to live quietly at home. In many cases this drug (and similar ones) has saved patients from undergoing electroshock therapy and other prolonged treatments in hospitals.

Of course, like any other drug, chlorpromazine is not a cure-all, but it certainly has its uses—especially in those who cannot sleep well because of mental aberrations requiring treatment. So don't listen to well-meaning neighbors who scare you with stories about the bad effects of drugs on the liver and blood. Your doctor is aware of any potential danger. He is on guard. Sometimes it comes down to a question of choosing the lesser of two evils (and chlorpromazine and similar drugs are far from being evils): watching a patient deteriorate or giving him a drug that may help him.

NO PLEA FOR SLEEPING PILLS

I suppose I should not be making a plea for the use of pills to promote relaxation and sleep in a country which spends at least 100 million dollars a year on some 350 tons of sleeping pills (that's a 400 per cent increase since 1935). Nevertheless, in spite of the thousands of cases in which pills are overused or incorrectly used, many patients require them for their use.

Barbiturates, hypnotics and sedatives are used, not only for insomnia, but also for those who suffer from high blood pressure, heart disease, epilepsy and convulsions and for those who live in stressful situations or are undergoing preparation for surgery. But their most important use is to prepare the patient for a good night's sleep. Doctors have a choice between scores of tried and trusted remedies such as Nembutal, Seconal, Amytal, chloral hydrate, paraldehyde and bromides. But the patient should take these drugs *only* under the supervision of a medical man.

Self-treatment is dangerous. Since drugs such as bromides can be bought over the counter without a doctor's prescription, the patient therefore gets a false feeling of security. "However much I take," he thinks, "it can't harm me." But he's wrong.

For example, if you take bromides every day, you are inviting an attack of bromidism: chronic bromide poisoning. It may cause skin eruptions, upset stomach, a cold that seems to hang on forever, loss of appetite and constipation. As the intoxication progresses, you may suffer from drowsiness, become completely disoriented, have hallucinations and lapse into unconsciousness and coma.

I have seen patients near death because their unconsciousness was at first attributed to something entirely different from bromide intoxication. If they hadn't had a blood bromide determination, they might have died. Treatment with salt solution and other remedies brought them back to life. The moral is clear: do not take any pills on your own, even though they are apparently harmless ones you can buy without a doctor's prescription.

Sleepmanship: Facts, Fiction, Fancies | III

16 | Sleep: Assorted Facts and Fiction

HERE IS A MEDICAL GRAB BAG of sleep information culled from experience in practice and many sources. Reach down deep and have some. You may come up with the very tidbit that will transform you from an insomniac into a welcome member of the brotherhood of the Land of Nod.

Try a cold-air bath in the nude; Ben Franklin used to do it.

To promote relaxation in the eyes try looking downward toward your toes until the eye muscles tire. They will then assume their upward sleeping position more readily.

You are a little taller in the morning than at night; your vertebrae settle during the day.

In susceptible persons eye strain may be a cause of insomnia.

We toss in bed whether we are worried or not, but we toss more if we are worried.

Women like to talk in their sleep, but not as much as men. According to one survey of hundreds of college students, 41 per cent of the males and 37 per cent of the females talked in their sleep.

Abe Lincoln liked to take a midnight walk as a preventative for insomnia.

You will not sleep well if your bed is too short or too narrow.

Sleeping schedules of night workers are usually erratic and unsatisfactory. When they get home at 8–9 A.M., they have breakfast and then go to sleep until about 1 P.M. Then they have lunch and another stretch of sleep for an hour or two. Many become irritable and wonder why. Chronic sleep loss is the answer.

If you have been taking tranquilizers or other sedatives, beware of "one for the road" just before taking the wheel. Alcohol and tranquilizers don't mix.

A person born blind does not "see" things in his dreams. His only dream sensations are those of touch, hearing and motion.

I have a friend who is cussing himself out as a fool. Although he has always been sensitive to noise, he has just bought an expensive home fronting on a main highway. "I haven't slept a wink since I live there. How foolish can a person get?"

The more an insomniac worries about how little sleep he is getting, the less he sleeps.

Muscles and mind stimulate each other.

The brain of the sleeping person receives more rather than less blood and oxygen. The old theory that we get sleepy because blood is drained from the brain is wrong.

One woman tried this variety of sleeping tips: bedtime snack; walk before bedtime; warm tub-bath; cold shower; electric blanket; cold compresses at the back of the neck. Nothing helped. One night she came upon the solution. "I went to bed wearing only scent-of-roses perfume. I've had no trouble sleeping since I started that habit."

I know a man who sleeps best when the foot of his bed is raised a few inches. But when the head of a puppy is lower than the rest of its body, it can't sleep well.

Married persons' life expectation is higher than that of those who remain single. Therefore, when your wife says, "You'll be the death of me with your snoring," don't become too apprehensive.

A nap in the sun may be enervating because much salt is lost through excessive sweating.

Don't be taken in by so-called experts who promise to interpret your dreams. You will find that they often also engage in palmistry, astrology, fortune-telling and other unproved methods of capturing the vagaries of the human mind.

A Chinese proverb states: "There is no economy in going to bed early to save candles if the result is twins."

Some persons require more sleep when they are old than when they were twenty years younger.

Insomnia is more likely to be found among brain workers than among physical workers.

Another name for insomnia is hyposomnia: a lessening of the duration and depth of sleep—one or both—lasting for a few nights or for weeks and months.

Considering our uterine beginnings, it is not surprising that many persons assume the fetal (curled up) attitude during sleep.

Aristotle compared wakefulness and sleep to health and disease: "For contraries, in natural as well as in other matters, are seen always to present themselves in the same subject, and to be affections of the same: examples are health and sickness, beauty and ugliness, strength and weakness, sight and blindness, hearing and deafness."

Where does drowsiness end and sleep begin? How often we say, "I don't remember just when I went to sleep."

Some people sleep so soundly that it is difficult to wake them; even water, noise or light has little effect. It seems that they somehow incorporate these interruptions into their dreams, thereby disguising them, and keep on sleeping.

Melancholic and depressed people frequently complain of waking early from sleep and feeling at their worst. Whenever patients come to me with this complaint, I try to discover what is really worrying them.

True or false? That older people need hardly any sleep? False. That one hour's sleep before midnight is worth two after? False.

There are three main classes of sleepers. The early-to-bed and early-to-rise type; the late-to-bed and late-to-rise type; and a type made of a mixture of the two. You should try to find your natural place on the seesaw between wakefulness and sleep.

Sleep has been rightly called "the original and natural tranquilizer."

Of the over 2,000 different barbitals that have been manufactured, doctors commonly use no more than a few dozen varieties.

Counting sheep may be a remedy for insomnia in some people, but I wonder if it doesn't keep as many awake. I believe it's how you count the sheep that matters. For example, I suggest you count the black sheep, or the sheep that jump the fence backwards, or the mother sheep looking for their lost youngsters.

Wives and husbands often ask, and wonder, why their partners are able to sleep so well while they have a nightly bout with insomnia. The answer, banal as it may seem, is that we are all different. Thus Joseph Breuer and Sigmund Freud wrote in their *Studies of Hysteria* that "the great differences between lively people and inert and lethargic ones, between those who 'cannot sit still' and those who have an 'innate gift for lounging on sofas' . . . are certainly based on profound differences in [the] nervous system."

The same differences explain, I believe, why some people can sleep through a violent thunderstorm while others are awakened by the drop of a pin.

A healthy man of eighty-five once told me that he had never slept in his entire life. That was the biggest whopper I had ever heard. He meant it, of course, but he was just one of those who are such light sleepers that they do not realize they have been asleep.

Many patients have told me that a half-hour nap after lunch is worth three hours of sleep at night. Such people are efficient catnappers.

The common belief that one cannot repay a sleep debt is untrue. If you have been up late night after night, you can liquidate the major portion of your debt in one good night's sleep.

I have a practical tip for men on how to beat undue fatigue. Take a lesson from the feminine sex. Whenever possible take off your shoes or, at least, loosen your laces. Do so at the theater, at the movies, on a long plane trip, while at home. It is surprising how much constriction of the feet contributes to tiredness. And remember, fatigue often prevents sleep.

According to Major Titov: "We cosmonauts have been trained by physicians to fall asleep instantly, when desired, and to wake up exactly at a given time." It is evident that some people require more training than others. Thus people should not give up too soon if they are unable to nap. Napping takes practice, and one doesn't have to be a cosmonaut to succeed.

Don't use heavy blankets. Remember that in an eight-hour sleep your breathing lifts the bedclothes at least 7,000 times.

Grown-ups do not fall out of bed at night because, even in sleep, they are aware of danger. I read recently of a young worker who took his after-lunch siesta high above the street on a girder. He did not fall, but I would not try it on a bet.

When stories about American prisoners' "squealing" in Korea reached this country, I could not understand why people reacted so violently. I think that Dr. Kleitman was right when he once said that however patriotic a man may be, he can get "to the point where he would confess anything just to be allowed to sleep." That is as true in peace as in war.

I wonder how many husbands and wives are frank enough to say: "I wish I had a big bed and room of my own."

According to one poll, 40 per cent of all women sleep nude; 25 per cent of all men. Of course, many sleep only in either pajama tops or pajama bottoms or in nightgowns. I know one fellow who sheepishly admitted he slept in a nightcap—nothing else.

My mother, until she died, aged eighty-two, swore by lettuce as the best hypnotic. However you get a good night's sleep—as long as the means is harmless—do not let your friends laugh you out of your method. One friend swears by buttered popcorn as a soporific.

An experiment that appears to prove that sleep is not due to a collection of fatigue-chemicals in the blood was conducted with Siamese twins who had an interconnecting circulation. While one remained very much awake, the other was often fast asleep.

Some people use a late dinner as a weapon against insomnia. They say that those who eat dinner at 5:30 P.M. and take nothing until the next morning are actually inviting insomnia. Others say that eating before bedtime or having a late dinner is sure to give them a restless night. *You* must be the judge of your own personal preferences and reactions.

Do not count up the lost hours of sleep, as some people do, and enter them in a diary. It isn't necessary to make up for every hour of lost sleep.

Night air is not dangerous, so open your windows if you wish. In fact, because of lessened traffic, night air may be less polluted and much cleaner than day air.

The average person goes to sleep in fifteen to twenty-five minutes. Many insomniacs become impatient and upset if they do not go to sleep immediately. The result of this impatience? More sleeplessness.

Laboratory mice have sixteen sleep periods. Horses have ten (one long one of about four hours, which they can take standing up). I do not advise horsenaps or mousenaps, but the catnap is almost essential to top efficiency.

In *Our Human Body* Ray Giles relates the story of Carl E. Seashore's discovery of the value of a nap at noon. Since then the famous psychologist has maintained that "fifteen minutes of sleep after the heaviest work and before the main meal count more for efficiency than five times as much late, light sleeping in the morning."

I think each of us can spare fifteen minutes a day, or more, for a nap. But, driven by some powerful force to "keep going," many of us will continue to live without forming the nap habit vital for putting some extra zing into our lives.

I have often found it to be true that the best night sedative, especially for the elderly, is an ounce of hard liquor, or an ounce or two of sherry, taken either with or without an aspirin tablet.

Frederic Damrau, M.D., Emma Liddy, B.A., and Adeline M. Damrau studied fifty-six otherwise healthy middle-aged or elderly persons having difficulty in sleeping. There were twenty-eight men and twenty-two women. Their ages ranged from thirty-five to eighty-five (average, 51.8 years). The insomnia was mild, moderate or severe.

The subjects were given a bottle (11.39 fluid ounces) of stout to drink before retiring and were told to report on drowsiness, quality of sleep and nocturia (the need to pass urine at night).

The researchers conclude that the consumption of one bottle of stout—one-sixth the amount required to produce an intoxicating level of alcohol in the blood—improved sleep in 76 per cent of the cases, did not improve it in 21 per cent of the cases and brought on a possible improvement in 3 per cent of the cases. "Stout apparently has a large field of application as a relaxing agent for the average person who has ordinary difficulties with sleeping. Its use in preference to sleeping pills obviates the danger of drug addiction and other untoward effects."

Many people think that sleep and hypnosis are the same, but it is not so. In hypnosis the typical brain-wave changes observed during normal sleep do not occur, the knee-jerk reflex still operates and the usual falls in blood pressure and pulse rate do not take place.

A good rule of thumb is that newborn babies require two hours of sleep for every one they are awake and adults require one hour of sleep for every two awake.

Though people may say they hear the clock strike every hour all night, you can be sure they couldn't hear them all week after week unless they slept between chimes.

For fatigue prevention, eat foods that contain glycogen and iron, the best fuel for muscles:

Carbohydrate foods furnishing glycogen: honey, molasses, sugar, beans, bread, crackers, oatmeal, dates, macaroni, rice, etc.

Foods high in iron: eggs, figs, lean beef, oatmeal, prunes, raisins, spinach, whole wheat, almonds, etc.

One of the common causes of insomnia is cerebral arteriosclerosis. Unfortunately, patients with this disease often react poorly to barbiturates. They become more confused and forgetful.

Deep breathing helps overcome tired feelings because oxygen acts on lactic acid to change it back to glycogen, a prime muscle food. Try deep breathing when you are too tired physically to go to sleep.

Fatigue may cause insomnia; insomnia may cause fatigue. Anxiety, which may cause people to think unceasingly during sleeping hours, can result in wakefulness. But it is also true that extreme happiness can also cause insomnia.

For a true insomniac a visit to Norman Dine's Sleep Center in New York City is an experience not unlike that of a child let loose in a large toy shop: there is such a varied assortment of sleep paraphernalia to choose from.

No part of the body ceases to function entirely during sleep.

Remember that chronic sleep loss is often the forerunner of a mental breakdown. Sleeplessness, like pain, should bring the patient to the doctor.

Don't wake fast; wake gradually. Watch the cat wake. Learn to stretch and yawn and get out of bed slowly. Especially if you are middle-aged or older, give your circulation a chance to catch up with the sudden change from inactivity to activity.

Everyone dreams: about one and one-half to two hours during an eight-hour sleep.

If you are concerned that naps taken during the day will interfere with the length and depth of your sleep at night, you may be relieved to know that they have no significant effect on a good night's sleep.

Always cover yourself when taking a nap, even in what appears to be a comfortably heated room. Otherwise you may wake stiff and chilled. Heat production drops off during sleep.

Tiredness, although often the friend of sleep, becomes its enemy if it turns into fatigue. An army marching for fifty minutes and resting for ten in each hour will cover more ground and be less fatigued at the end of eight hours than if it marches for three hours and twenty minutes, then rests for eighty minutes, then marches again for three hours and twenty minutes. Therefore, in home or office, try to interrupt what you are doing every fifty minutes (use an alarm clock, if necessary) for a short break.

According to R. Kingman: "Those who sleep eight hours and believe that they need 10 consider themselves to be suffering just as much from insomnia as others who cannot get more than 4–5 hours of sleep but who would be satisfied with six or seven."

Cervantes said: "May blessing light upon him who first invented sleep! It is food for the hungry, drink for the thirsty, heat for the cold, and cold for the hot. It is the coin that buys all things, and the balance that makes the king even with the shepherd, and the fool with the wise." (Ask any insomniac.)

One practical way to do away with worries is to keep a pad and pencil at your bedside and to write down what's worrying you about yesterday's or tomorrow's problems. This often resolves anxieties, or lessens them, and permits sleep.

"Leg cramps" is a common complaint in insomnia. You go to sleep feeling fit and looking forward to a good night's sleep. Suddenly you are awakened by a grip of steel around the calf of a leg. Immediately you think, what would have happened if this came on while I was swimming. You massage it for a moment or two, but it doesn't help. So you hop out of bed and walk around until it disappears. It may happen once in ten years or ten times in one month. The cause? We don't know. The treatment? Many have been helped by taking a five-grain quinine pill before bedtime.

If these cramps occur in the aging and are paralleled by attacks of leg pain on exertion, then a complete review of the leg circulation is imperative to rule out serious artery or vein disease in the legs.

Dr. M.M. Miller found that merely eliminating excess salt from the diet relieved some severe cases of insomnia.

Hiatal (diaphragmatic) hernia is a cause of sleeplessness. In this condition some smaller or greater part of the abdominal contents (stomach, etc.) has slipped up into the chest through an abnormal enlargement in the diaphragm—a hernial opening. This causes difficulty in breathing and sometimes actual chest pain, which has occasionally been confused with a coronary attack. A simple trick to overcome the discomfort is to sleep on three or four pillows. If you sleep flat, gravity itself has a tendency to allow the abdominal contents to slip into the chest. In addition, those who have this trouble should not overburden the stomach with a heavy meal at night. Sedatives and relaxants will help them sleep well. Operation should be considered only after a long trial at conservative treatment.

Among the elderly Parkinson's disease and hypertrophy of the prostate are common causes of disturbed sleep. About 25 per cent of the patients with Parkinson's disease have difficulty in sleeping. As many drugs are used in the treatment of this chronic ailment to reduce tremor and promote relaxation of the muscles, the doctor will try various combinations to find the one best suited to each individual patient. In spite of the best of care, sleep can be a chronic problem for the Parkinson patient: he either sleeps very well or badly. His best hours are often between 7 A.M. and 1 P.M.

Patients with prostate trouble have to get up several times at night to urinate because of the irritation caused by enlarged prostate on the neck of the urinary bladder. Consequently, insomnia in such patients is often cured by the urologic surgeon. If the prostate is large, chances are that massage of the prostate will not help the patient get over his frequent urination. When faced with the need for operation, the elderly insomniac should not hesitate simply because he is in his seventies or eighties. Many such patients withstand surgery as well as younger men. What counts is not so much calendar age as the physiological age of the patient. Some arteries in seventy-year-old patients are younger than those in men of fifty.

Heart attacks and strokes may occur during sleep, which isn't always the restful state people think it is. Some patients have been awakened with an angina attack because of the stress encountered in a nightmare. How often have you awakened from a disturbing dream with a pounding heart?

It is good policy not to go to sleep with a greatly disturbed mind. An emotional binge before sleep is inviting trouble for the high blood pressure sufferer or for the coronary patient. Take a good tranquilizer and settle down before retiring.

Often, suggestion will produce sleep where everything else fails. I have a simple prescription that may put you in the mood for sleep. Repeat slowly and distinctly Joseph Devlin's synonyms for sleep, and you may soon have to close your eyes and surrender to Morpheus: "slumber, doze, drowse, nap, snooze, hibernate, dream, snore, nod, yawn, languish, flag, relax, go to bed, rest in the arms of Morpheus, close the eyelids, hit the hay."

Try it sometimes.

One important reason for not taking steadily increasing doses of barbiturates without a doctor's supervision is the danger of withdrawal symptoms when you decide to give them up. Sometimes the symptoms are severe enough to cause psychotic delirium or convulsions.

The successful are usually good sleepers. Thornton Wilder once wrote: "I could sleep on a heap of shoes."

People love to talk about sleep. Next to a discussion about the weather, what is more commonly heard than "How'd you sleep last night?"

We don't "waste time" sleeping.

Rube Goldberg said he could not sleep without a pillow on his feet.

Ask a farmhand about insomnia, and he will say, "What's that?"

When we sleep, we revert to our primitive selves. Thus we always sleep "on guard."

"Sleep comes not to him who is cold, nor to him who is hungry, not to him who is in fear"—Arab proverb.

"Whilst Adam slept Eve from his side arose: strange his first sleep should be his last repose"—Anon.

"Bed is your brother"—Swahili saying.

"Sleep, like the Kingdom of Heaven, is not taken by force"—Bolton Hall.

In *The Pickwick Papers*, Mr. Wardle's fat boy Joe just ate and slept; he was probably a narcoleptic. From him we get the term Pickwickian syndrome.

". . . and if, for a while, I could give her rest and sleep, she would be a new woman"—Dr. Walter Alvarez.

"Blessed are the sleepy, for they shall soon drop off"—Nietzsche.

"Never go to bed with cold feet, or a cold heart"—William Hone (1841).

I have some justification for my mother's belief in the therapeutic actions of lettuce leaf. William Vaughn (1602) wrote to Galen: "He was faine to eat boyled lettice, with a little butter at the end of his supper, when he was old."

If you are now twenty, you will sleep for about another sixteen and one-half years. If you are now forty, you will sleep for about another ten years. If you are now sixty, you will sleep for about another three and one-half years.

"I wonder if anyone ever counts sheep in a spot like this? I can't even stand the sight of mutton. The smell of lamb chop turns my stomach. I've tried the hot milk and the tepid bath. Nothing works"—Jimmy Cannon.

Nursing puppies will die within a week if denied sleep. They could go a month without food without dying.

Lack of sufficient sleep results in less control of emotions: pessimism replaces cheerfulness and irritability supersedes philosophical calm.

"Sleeplessness is a curse as old as man himself. . . . It seems to resist the wheedlings of progress; indeed its prevalence increases in step with life's growing complexity. . . . It likes to be courted and can only be seduced under conditions which are perfectly in keeping with its mood"—John and Diana St. John.

"The precept of 'trying to go to sleep,' commonly recommended to children and invalids, is one of the most silly that ever gained currency by language. 'To sleep' is not an active verb; and sleeping is not an active function. Any sort of mental activity, the resolve 'to do' for example, is unfavorable to the result and therefore retards it"—*The Leisure Hour* (1865).

Until recently at least, sleeping in barber shops was unlawful in Buffalo, N.Y.

I am not certain where they originated, but I have a hunch that "teaching records" are an American invention. Only those who have tried to put the "wasted hours" of sleep to good use would ever think of inventing language records with mikes under the sleeper's pillow so he could learn a new language while sleeping.

From what I hear, investigation of results has disclosed that the high hopes of these unconscious students have not materialized as well as expected. In other words, the old-fashioned way of learning is still a necessity: you have to stay awake!

Drs. Charles W. Simon and William H. Emmons, who studied sleep-teaching at the RAND Corporation, Santa Monica, California, concluded their report by saying that "learning during sleep is impractical and probably impossible." However, it is possible that some degree of learning may take place "during a marginal, waking state."

"Lack of sleep in itself is a stress"—Dr. Hans Selye.

Animals when deprived of sleep become vicious.

According to a recent survey, 52 per cent of all adults suffer from some degree of insomnia. (The other 48 per cent do not sympathize or understand.)

Dr. Charles Fisher, psychiatrist of Mt. Sinai Hospital, New York, said: "The dream is the normal psychosis—dreaming permits each of us to be quietly and safely insane every night of our lives."

The brain needs sleep much more than the muscles.

The average yawn is seldom due to boredom; rather, it is a physiological answer to the need for more oxygen—often expressed when suffering from fatigue, hunger, indigestion or poor ventilation. The yawn simply reinforces ordinary respiration.

Incidentally, Darwin observed that baboons reveal hostility by yawning. (Is yawning, then, an unconscious sign of some listeners' hostility to speakers?)

It does not matter whether you sleep on your left side or on your right because you change your position thirty to forty times a night.

It does not injure your heart to sleep on your left side for a greater or shorter time.

17 | Bedside Advice from Readers

MONTHS AGO I sent out a distress signal to readers of my newspaper column. I felt that this book would not be complete unless I incorporated some first-hand experiences in fighting insomnia.

In part, I wrote in the column:

> Getting a good night's sleep may not be easy. What works for one doesn't for his next-door neighbor. What I'd like you to do is to send me a letter which states your problem.
>
> Is it snoring? Inability to fall asleep? Inability to stay asleep? Wakefulness in early morning hours? Or any one of a score of other complaints?
>
> Out of this practical "research" may come an inkling, at least, of the answer. We have learned much about the mechanics of sleep and dreams through the investigations of scientists in their laboratories, but further study of thousands of personal sleep problems by such a poll as this may offer some additional important clues.
>
> If you have suffered from insomnia and have overcome it, please tell me how. If snoring no longer keeps your family awake within a radius of 25 yards, tell me how you accomplished the miracle.
>
> Call them tricks, tips or what you will; send them on. They may add up to something useful. Consider yourself as participating in a scientific experiment by writing about your personal experiences.
>
> During the past few years I have been doing some se-

rious investigation into the sleep problem. With your help, perhaps I can come up with some simple suggestion here and there which will provide the balm of sleep to insomniacs who have practically given up; who think they will never again experience the sweet surcease and satisfaction of a good night's sleep.

At least we can try. Anything's better than turning and tossing night after night in hopeless surrender to insomnia.

In answer to this request I have received letters from all over the United States and Canada. As there is insufficient space to include them all, I have made abstracts from the most provocative and helpful and include them here. Somewhere, somehow one or more of these tips from fellow-sufferers may be your key to locking the door against wakefulness.

Dear Dr. Steincrohn:

I have suffered from insomnia at irregular intervals over the past ten years. My solution is a couple of small cocktails before bed with an occasional sleeping pill. Otherwise I do not drink.

Dear Dr. Steincrohn:

If anybody should have insomnia, I should. I had a lung removed almost five years ago. I can't walk without getting short of breath. But I am able to work as a carpenter, and I still get a good night's sleep. I let my problems stay at work and don't get into bed with them. Speaking of bed, I've always believed in a good one. Seven years ago I bought myself a bed that cost $115.00. It's the best buy I ever made.

Dear Dr. Steincrohn:

For people who want help to overcome sleepless nights this is the most: take a warm bath, then lie in bed thinking of the nice things of the day. Start taking deep breaths slowly, in and out. Ten of them and you'll be in dreamland.

Dear Dr. Steincrohn:

For many years I've listened to soft music on the radio; I found I could rest quietly even if I didn't sleep well.

Dear Dr. Steincrohn:

Re insomnia. I've found that limiting my coffee intake to one cup per meal, eliminating it between meals and taking none with the evening meal helps much. Also it is relaxing to take a hot sitz bath at bedtime; keep the water temperature as hot as you can stand it. After fifteen minutes of this you will be relaxed and pleasantly exhausted and hardly able to wait to sleep. Also, it is good to remember that when you are in bed, you are getting 75 per cent of your needed rest, and that worrying about not sleeping will keep you awake. The 25 per cent you are going to lose through wakefulness is not going to harm you anyway.

Dear Dr. Steincrohn:

For years (I am now thirty-seven) I would toss and turn and have a terrible time going to sleep. It would take me two to three hours at least. The next day I was so pooped I could lie down on the sofa early in the afternoon and drop off to sleep immediately. I always tried to console myself by saying that I had an active mind and couldn't calm it down at night or that my husband snored or with some such excuse.

Then four years ago I discovered what caused my sleepless nights when *I quit smoking*. I had never smoked much in the morning, but in the late afternoon and evening I really smoked a lot. This may sound fantastic, but I think your readers ought to know that I haven't had one sleepless night since! I go to bed now knowing I'll drop off immediately; I don't even stay awake long enough to hear my husband snore.

I'll wager that thousands of people who have been searching years for a solution to their insomnia problems have never even considered the possibility that smoking may be the cause. I know I didn't even suspect it until I quit.

Dear Dr. Steincrohn:

I find that the world's best short stories and essays, culled by many specialists, are good volumes to have at your bedside. Rather than abuse yourself with thoughts that will not control themselves, it is better to pick up one of these volumes. Jot down on it the time of your first yawn, which is the psychological moment to slide well under your electric blanket into deep sleep.

Dear Dr. Steincrohn:

I have three methods of wooing sleep, and I like all equally well.

1. I fit a soft pillow into the hollow of my neck. Then I relax completely, making my body as heavy as possible. I begin counting backwards from one hundred to one, taking a rather deep breath between counts. You can't

think of anything else if you persist in counting slowly and regularly. If I falter, I start again at one hundred. I am soon asleep.

2. Forget "me." I read somewhere that we think of ourselves 90 per cent of our waking hours: *our* friends, *our* money matters, *our* social life. I know I begin thinking such thoughts the minute I hit the bed. So I stop thinking of myself; instead, I think of the universe, the astronauts; about the rest of our great country; about what other families are doing; about people dancing and having fun. Sometimes I think of food—where coffee, tea, fruit, beef, fish, etc., are grown and processed. I think of the north and south poles and wonder how anyone can live in such cold. Keeping your mind away from "me" works, believe me.

3. I purchased a transistor radio not long ago, and I dearly love to listen to restful music. I keep the volume low and the soothing music gradually lulls me to sleep. When I wake to change position, I sometimes turn the radio off. But just as often I settle down to listen again.

Dear Dr. Steincrohn:

I don't think one lies awake consciously, but I do think that too often folks go to bed with the idea firmly established that they won't be able to sleep. Consequently, they toss and fret while they *work* at getting to sleep.

You hear folks say, "I can't drink coffee at night. I would not sleep a wink." Why is it so terrible to lie awake at night? One can lie there and rest and relax and think—unless one tries too hard and frets too much about loss of sleep.

There are several reasons for sleeplessness. Heavy eating before bedtime is one. Being too cold or too hot is another. Occasionally, there is no apparent reason.

If I'm cold, I take measures to insure warmth. If I'm comfortable but still can't sleep, I may read. If my eyes are already tired, I simply lie there and think. I find that prayer always helps me quiet down. So does reciting scripture and poetry. Fighting to get to sleep will get one nowhere. I am seventy-three now, so I should know.

Dear Dr. Steincrohn:

As a registered nurse who has specialized in pediatrics, I would like to add my bit to the "insomnia research project" that you have invited us to join.

A baby sleeps well if his stomach is comfortable, that is, if the formula agrees with him. If he has colic, he lets everyone know about his discomfort. I really believe that many cases of insomnia are due to stomach discomfort, that is, to eating wrong foods before bedtime or to eating when nervous, tense and overtired.

Of course, arthritic pain will keep one awake, as will any other pain or discomfort for that matter. We cannot place all insomnia cases in the same category. Personally, if I cannot sleep (and I usually do sleep well), I take an antacid or drink a half-glass of warm milk. Then I say the 91st Psalm over to myself. If I am still awake, I count my blessings and pray. Usually, I have dropped off in a refreshing sleep in a short time.

Dear Dr. Steincrohn:

If you are wakeful in the early morning hours, you probably did not eat enough at the evening meal. Get up and drink some milk (not too cold) or eat a light meal of cereal and fruit.

Dear Dr. Steincrohn:

Re the snoring problem. Sleep in a separate bed and have a proper mattress and springs. Be thankful for the snorer; think how unhappy you would be if he or she were not there. Then you will be in a mood to sleep no matter how loud the snoring.

Dear Dr. Steincrohn:

One summer years and years ago my parents and I slept in a small cabin, roughing it. We had bunks in the same room, and they both snored. If I could get to sleep first, I was O.K. But when I didn't . . . !

One night in exasperation I reached for a newspaper. I was going to throw balls of paper at them. But when the noise of the ripping paper cracked the silence, they both stopped. After that, that was all that I had to do: tear up a newspaper. The only trouble was that it kept me up, too.

Dear Dr. Steincrohn:

I have a simple insomnia cure. It has worked for me and for a few friends who have tried it. I lie on my back, place a hot-water bottle on my stomach and lay the inside of my wrists on it. Away I go.

Dear Dr. Steincrohn:

A smart program manager of a radio station would start a sleep program: music, talk, recitations, etc. It's purpose would not be to keep the listener interested and awake; instead, it would be to make him bored and sleepy. The first station that tried it would have a hit on its hands.

Dear Dr. Steincrohn:

My husband is a teeth-grinder. For years I prayed for the day when he'd need false teeth so he would take them out at night and let me sleep. It does no good to leave the bedroom as the infernal noise can be heard all over the house. But a year ago a wonderful dentist came up with the solution. He made my husband a thin transparent plate that fits over his upper teeth. Now he grinds to his heart's content and doesn't make a sound. It's such a pleasure to lie down and just drift peacefully off to sleep.

Dear Dr. Steincrohn:

I get complete relief for my restless legs by raising them perpendicularly to my body. While lying on my back I slide my feet up the wall until both my legs make a right angle with my body. Simple, but it works.

Dear Dr. Steincrohn:

I cured my restless legs by wearing extra arch supports in my shoes.

Dear Dr. Steincrohn:

Some years ago, in desperation, I tried a homemade version of a whirlpool bath for my restless legs. I sit on the edge of the tub with feet and ankles under the faucet and turn on the water full force. I alternate the hot and cold for about ten minutes and finish off with an alcohol rub. I get to sleep without any further difficulty.

Dear Dr. Steincrohn:

For months I used to be unable to sleep at least one week in four. My doctor finally diagnosed premenstrual tension. He has given me hormones and a drug to remove excess water from my system, and I now sleep like a baby.

Dear Dr. Steincrohn:

I have no difficulty falling asleep. My trouble shows up sometime after 3 A.M. Sometimes I wake up and cannot go back to sleep at all. Sometimes I just wake up and doze for the remainder of the night. I have unpleasant dreams and many nightmares. The next day I feel miserable.

The cure, if you can call it that, is taking one sleeping pill per night. On doctor's orders. That does the trick. I have been doing it for years.

Dear Dr. Steincrohn:

As a former insomniac I'll add my remedy to that of your other readers. I'm a woman in my early thirties with three children, so I'm tired at night. Sleep and nightmares have been a problem for about fifteen years, off and on. Looking back over the remedies I've tried there's only one that has really worked: relieving tension.

When I don't come to a climax with my husband, I stay awake most of the night because I am so tense. My insomnia however is a thing of the past since my husband and I have taken the trouble to make sexual "timing" a must in our household.

Dear Dr. Steincrohn:

Here is my cure for insomnia: quiet thinking. I take a thought such as "relax" or "God" and think it over and over. This way I rest and refresh my brain and fall asleep. Then there's another way: self-hypnosis. Keep saying to yourself, "I am *so* sleepy, I am *so* sleepy." Keep your mind on this, and you will soon be asleep.

Dear Dr. Steincrohn:

For many years I was troubled with insomnia, but now I have no more sleepless nights. Prayer releases all my tension, and I sleep.

Sleepmanship: Practical Methods | IV

18 | The Basic Strategy for Overcoming Insomnia

DR. SAMUEL JOHNSON said, "A man . . . afflicted [with insomnia] must divert distressing thoughts and not combat with them. To attempt to *think them down* is madness.

"He should have a lamp constantly burning in his bed chamber during the night, and if wakeful or disturbed, take a book and read, and compose himself to rest. To have the management of the mind is a great art, and it may be attained in a considerable degree by experience and habitual exercise."

So if you have insomnia, the first practical pointer is: don't lie there staring into the darkness. Get up. Do something. I have a friend who gets up to shave at 3 A.M. This gives him such a feeling of satisfaction (knowing he will not have to shave in the morning) that he falls right off to sleep. I've heard of a man who wrote a novel he had worked at during two years of sleepless nights.

One insomniac knows the value of this:

Dear Dr. Steincrohn:

It is 3 A.M. and, as usual, I am unable to sleep. So I thought it might be a good time to tell you of my various attempts to overcome insomnia.

I am forty-five years old and for the past five years I have been plagued with this maddening handicap while my dear husband gets eight hours of uninterrupted sleep and could probably go on for ten, given the chance. My one child, a teen-aged daughter, has no sleeping problem, so I prowl about much of the night in lonely splendor.

I have tried many methods of overcoming my affliction but all without success. Even pills have failed me.

I have therefore decided to relax and enjoy what little sleep I can get, using the rest of the night for something else. When you come right down to it, doesn't it seem pretty silly to try to force myself to get eight-hours-or-so sleep when I can manage on four?

The trouble seems to be that only relaxed people can learn to relax, and they don't need lessons. The tense types, like myself, are the ones who need to relax, and we simply can't. The more we work at relaxing the more tense we get. It's a vicious circle. Yet the only way I've licked insomnia is by thumbing my nose at it.

True, it is hard to learn to relax. But with patience it is possible, as Dr. Edmund Jacobson shows in his well-known book *You Must Relax*. It may take 150 hours of instruction and twice that many hours of practice to be able to relax at will any muscles of the body, but you *can* do it.

To be able to relax each muscle, you must learn how to "de-stretch" yourself by means of "progressive relaxation." As you gradually relax first your legs, then your back and abdomen, and then your shoulders and arms, you become limp, a dead weight. The muscles of your jaw and neck are often the last to let go. By that time you are asleep or close to it. The best way to fall asleep remains to forget about falling asleep, but if you can't do that, try progressive relaxation.

TOO MUCH OR NOT ENOUGH?

Alexis Carrel wrote that man must learn to control all his drives, including "his need of sleep. Modern man sleeps too much or not enough. He does not easily adapt himself in this respect. It is useful to accustom oneself to remain awake when one wants to sleep. The struggle against sleep sets in motion organic apparatuses whose strength develops by exercise." In other words, such exercises develop the will.

Too much or not enough? Carrel has made an important point there.

The answer lies in how you feel the next morning. Do you get up tired or sufficiently rested? Is getting out of bed a test of willpower, or do you jump out as if you have been released from bondage? How do you feel in the afternoon? Drowsy? Or energetic?

Each one of us must make his own evaluation. No doctor can do it for you, and I certainly don't propose to try. But it is important to know in which category you belong. If you really need eight or nine hours a night and have been getting only six, then the lack of sleep is bound to catch up with you, either in your work efficiency or in your capacity to enjoy life.

On the other hand, if you need only six hours of rest at night and stay in bed for nine hours because you've heard "it's good for you," then you will just be wasting three hours in every twenty-four just as surely as you would be wasting money scattering ten dollar bills into the wind. Time is more important than money. And for most people, sleep is so special that they would not think of trading it for any amount of money.

SOME PRACTICAL SUGGESTIONS

Sleep may be a matter of the mind for those who, sleeping badly, are still able to stay awake the next day. But how about the millions of us who are asleep on our feet after a night-long bout with insomnia? If it is in the mind, how do we overcome sleeplessness?

Our first practical suggestion is based on the theory that the control centers that regulate sleep and wakefulness are two small parts of the brain stem: the "reticular formation" and the "hypothalamus." Since these centers are constantly being bombarded by messages, some sensitive individuals might therefore sleep better if they were to make their bedrooms soundproof and lightproof. This, of course, is an extreme remedy, but some persons require such methods to overcome insomnia.

Ordinarily, insomnia is caused by the inability to relax, so try to think "loose." Your muscles are often tight and tense when you think they are relaxed. Make sure that your eyes are not tense. Try to make the lids as heavy as if actual weights were placed upon them. Open your mouth so that your lips become loosened and slack.

When you are awake in bed, your thoughts keep racing. You are thinking about family problems, business and personal worries, husband, wife, children, parents, friends and things that you did or didn't do. Consequently, your job is to try to substitute calm thoughts for these sleep-disturbers. Think of the times when you were fishing or paddling a canoe, lying in a garden or relaxing on a long trip.

The fear of insomnia is the greatest and most disturbing

worry. It is the thoughts of how tired you are surely going to be tomorrow because of the loss of sleep tonight and the fear of not falling asleep and staying asleep that cause much insomnia. Worrying about insomnia and its results makes you more tense, and there the vicious circle begins again. If you can only convince yourself that even after a sleepless night you will somehow get through the next day, that such loss of sleep will not cause your vital organs to sustain permanent damage, that "it doesn't matter," insomnia will soon be saying good-bye permanently.

Many have been able to neutralize their insomnia by taking time to prepare for bed. Try to cut down on your thinking at least a half-hour before retiring. Eliminate all thoughts of business. Leisurely choose your clothes for the next day. Take a hot bath, if baths usually make you relax. If you like to read, make a habit of reading a little before turning out the light. Some recommend hard reading to make the eyelids heavy; others, like William Saroyan, prefer pleasurable reading.

SUGGESTIONS BY INSOMNIACS

However you do it—and some even do it by allowing themselves to daydream—you must relax before and while you go to bed.

Thus one patient wrote:

> Years ago I found that concern, whether conscious or unconscious, was a great handicap to sleep. If concern turns to fear, all is lost. Bedtime should be thought of as a time for sweet peace, comfort and relaxation after the

cares of the day. Whatever tomorrow brings can be dealt with then. (In any case, things probably won't be as bad as they are imagined in the stillness of the night.)

Prayer has worked miracles for many insomniacs. Here is a letter from a woman who has never known what it is to suffer from loss of sleep:

> I have never had insomnia and would like to pass on to you my secrets.
>
> First, I believe in making the bedroom as attractive and the bed as comfortable as possible. I believe the best mattress you can afford is a good investment, and clean sheets and pillow cases and the proper covering and room temperature are important.
>
> Second, I think the mind must be prepared for sleep. I do this through sincere prayer to God. Almost immediately my worries of the day, and I have many, seem to fly away, and I am asleep before I really finish my prayer. I sleep soundly all night. I awake in the morning feeling refreshed.
>
> I am fifty-two years old, married and have a family. I'm not what you might call a deeply religious person, but my little private prayer does wonders for me.

WEEKEND SLEEPLESSNESS

Quite a few people become depressed, anxious and sleepless on weekends. At work or involved in the usual routine of the week, they are well-adjusted and happy. On Friday night, Saturday and Sunday, however, they get the blues. They are unhappy and sleepless; life loses its flavor. They can't understand why. "Hanging around" waiting for their regular week to begin becomes more than deadly boredom. They speak of it as an actual pain in the psyche.

I have found that such persons are not necessarily psychoneurotic. Many fall into a class you and I would call normal human beings. It seems that something in everyone resists change. We are wound up and tense to meet and overcome the problems that arise during the work-a-day week, and suddenly the brakes are applied. Our regular momentum is brought to a quick halt. Our minds are still racing, but our bodies are suspended. Thus it is our inability to adjust quickly from work to inactivity that causes weekend insomnia.

The remedy is evident. Guard against inactivity on the weekend. Plan ahead. Know on Monday what you are going to do on Friday night and all day Saturday and Sunday. Don't spend the weekend dawdling around the house, wondering why you have the blues. Hikes, picnics, visiting, golf, seeing people—these take up the slack in activity. But vary your schedule: visit different people. The key to successful weekend living is to keep up your momentum but in an entirely different way.

Boredom, blues and insomnia are often synonymous. Some are more susceptible to this weekend change than others. If you get the weekend blues, try these practical suggestions and you may find that the blue days turn rose-colored.

Many people suffer from sleep loss because they are "sleep-cheats." They can sleep but they won't. Either they don't go to sleep early enough or they are neurotic and afraid to go to sleep. (Of course, some can sleep two three-hour spells in twenty-four hours and feel as fresh as those who sleep eight hours. Perhaps this is the reason so many moonlighters seem to thrive, although few actually do.)

Often the clue to insomnia may be found in a review of the preceding day: food, naps, work, smoking, drinking, type of recreation and exercise, state of health, time of retiring and collateral factors. Basically, the cause of lost sleep is emotional when physical illness is not the predominant cause.

It has been said that "one man's lullaby is another man's insomnia." Does the neighbor's blaring radio or TV keep you awake? I have a friend who thrives on the noise; he goes to sleep with a smile. On nights when it is quiet, he wrestles with insomnia. He now has at his bedside an automatic radio to bring him the cacophony of sound he desires.

Does noisy plumbing keep you awake? Many have told me that the drip, drip, drip of a leaky faucet was as sleep-productive as the sound of gently falling rain.

Street noises? You have probably heard about the man from New York City who went to the country for two weeks and suffered interminable insomnia. He said the "quiet" kept him awake.

Does your husband's snoring keep you awake? Many women have confided in me that they slept less when their snoring husband was away on a business trip than when they heard the reassuring evidence of his presence in the house.

Crying children? How many of you whose children are grown and married sleep as well as you did when they lived at home and filled the house with little and big problems?

Does your partner insist on a double bed? Is he a restless sleep robber? Many women (and men) say: "I can't sleep well alone."

INSOMNIA ATTACKS ON MANY FRONTS

And so it goes. Insomnia attacks on all fronts and vanquishes the strong as well as the weak. It comes in many guises, but the effect is the same: threshing about, restlessness, worry about the morrow and a complete depression about life in general as you lie there trying to catch up on lost sleep.

Too much coffee or cola drinks? Leg cramps? Restless legs? Headache? Eating cheese before bedtime? Constipation? Heart skips? Itching rectum? Cold feet? Hay fever? A chronic cough? Prostate trouble? Diarrhea? A fear of dying? Nightmares? Whatever the reason or reasons, insomnia is a problem that should engage the full attention of your doctor. When you visit him, tell him all about it. Too many patients think it is a silly complaint in a world filled with cancer, heart disease and deadly accidents. But it *is* important. And no doctor should laugh it off lightly.

19 | Practical Pointers for Overcoming Insomnia

FEW PEOPLE ARE BORN WITH the ability to relax. Most of us have to learn how to do it through constant practice. And to do that, you must *want* to learn. Otherwise, you will go through life tense and unhappy.

If you are tense, you should first have a complete physical examination to make certain that the tenseness is not caused by illness, such as overactive thyroid gland, deep-seated anxieties, high blood pressure, etc., for all illnesses can cause tenseness.

But let us suppose that you are healthy. Then it's a matter of learning how to relax. The most important thing to learn is how to become a "snoozer." I have already discussed this, but the subject is so important to your well-being that it bears repeating that a snooze after lunch, a snooze before dinner at night, a Sunday afternoon snooze—all snoozes made a part of your daily schedule help eliminate tension and make up for lost sleep.

At first snoozes won't come easily. It may take months before you learn to snooze at the drop of a hat. But then the first months of scratchy violin practice don't sound like music. You reap the benefits of any sort of practice only after weeks and weeks of applying yourself to the job in hand.

When I transform a tense person into a snoozer, I know I am doing a good job for my patient. Snoozing has helped many an ulcer, coronary and high blood pressure patient more than medicine. Some of my most grateful patients have been those whom I taught how to snooze. Try it. See if it isn't the number one antidote against tension and the greatest defense against insomnia.

I have found that the one who naps every day rarely complains about loss of sleep at night even if he suffers from insomnia. In fact, many insomniacs have said that learning to nap has helped them feel sufficiently relaxed to sleep better.

Chauncey M. Depew would take a nap before attending an evening banquet. Stephens College in Missouri urged its 600 girl students to nap from 1–2 P.M. Result: faculty reported scholastic improvement.

Other famed nappers include General MacArthur and Presidents Truman, Eisenhower, Kennedy and Johnson. The elder Rockefeller benefitted from his daily snoozes. Mothers of many young children have learned how much revitalization the daily nap can induce.

According to William Kitay's book, *The Challenge of Medicine*: "Tension increases as the day goes on . . . if the business executive breaks it at noon with a short nap the tension curve drops to near the base line, and he awakens for the work of the afternoon, refreshed."

Winston Churchill made a ritual out of napping, advising that the best way to make the most of a nap is to undress and nap in a darkened room. This practice enabled him to work late into the night and be fresh for his many conferences. And his method is preferable to catching a quick nap in an armchair, for complete relaxation is possible only when lying down.

In his *The Character and the Conduct of Life*, William McDougall, M.B., F.R.S., wrote: "For people past middle life, the practice of sleeping for a short time in the afternoon is much to be recommended, especially if they do not enjoy long, sound sleep at night," for it both improves their performance in the evening and, if not carried to excess, "conduces to better sleep at night."

McDougall also says that napping gives women better health and helps preserve their looks, but that few women use it as a health- and beauty-aid.

DO NOT REFUSE SLEEPING PILLS

I have known many patients to go from day to day feeling like martyrs because they refuse to take sleeping pills, even when prescribed by their doctor. "It's dope," they say. "Not for me. I don't want to get into the habit of taking the stuff."

I have had to argue long and hard to get some insomniacs to take sleeping pills, if only for a few nights, to break up a dangerous cycle of sleeplessness, for, as I have said, protracted loss of sleep is often one of the first indications of a severe nervous collapse.

Patients won't go wrong if they take these medicines only under the advice of their physician. If he says take pills, then I advise you to take them. You will get into trouble only if you bootleg pills. When the prescription has run out, do not attempt to get it refilled without your doctor's knowledge. You will never get into the habit of taking sleeping pills if you follow this rule. Think of sleeping pills as temporary crutches to get you over some rough spots in life. Unless you are the type who overdoes in everything—oversmokes, overdrinks, overworks, etc.—I doubt that you will ever be in the position to describe your reliance on sleep pills as a dope habit.

All people who smoke are not chain-smokers; all people who drink are not chronic alcoholics; all people who take sleeping pills are not addicts.

Nevertheless, I am aware that the indiscriminate use of sleeping pills (even of tranquilizers) is potentially dangerous and can result in anything from the habitual use of a pill or two every night for years to the ultimate danger, suicide. But I tell people that where drugs are concerned, all is not black or white, bad or good. There are many gray areas where the pills act as necessary aids to get people over difficult periods of stress.

For example, consider Mr. H., aged forty-eight:

> I'm exhausted and at the end of my rope. I've been worried sick by financial losses and family worries and sickness. As a result, I haven't been able to sleep for months. My doctor told me weeks ago to take a sleeping pill every night for a while so that I could get at least some relief, but I have refused to take them. I've heard they're dope and that you can become an addict.

This man's eyes were red-rimmed and black-circled. He had lost about twenty pounds in weight. His hands shook, and he smoked cigarette after cigarette. He drank fifteen to twenty cups of black coffee every day "to keep going."

At last I convinced him that if he followed directions, he would not become an addict; that if he didn't get some rest right away, he would be inviting trouble much worse than addiction to sleeping pills. He agreed to take a barbiturate every night, as directed. Within ten days he had regained a half-dozen pounds and had cut down his coffee and cigarette intake to respectable amounts. He was being overdramatic when he said, "Those pills saved my life," but many patients have felt similar relief.

I agree that if you get into the habit of popping pills into your mouth at night as if they were so much hard candy, you court disaster. But so do you if you speed in your car, drink too much, smoke too much. Does it make good sense to dismiss sleeping pills because a few people abuse their use? Think of how much they help millions of others. You will never go far wrong if you follow these rules:

Never hesitate to take sleeping pills if your doctor thinks you need them. Some of my patients have taken a nightly pill for many years with beneficial, not harmful, results.

Never take sleeping pills on your own prescription. (Sometimes a neighbor or friend will let you have some his own doctor has prescribed. However well-intentioned, these people are dope "pushers.")

Never bootleg sleeping pills. Once your doctor's prescription has been used up, don't try to get a refill by devious means.

Never keep a full bottle of pills at your bedside table.

Never take sleeping pills after a night of drinking. Pills and alcohol don't mix.

Husband and wife should not take sleeping pills on the same night to guard against fire or burglary.

Do not take pills the night before a long car drive.

Sleeping pills or sedatives can cause havoc in the aged, who may become confused and act as if they are out in "left field."

Never give your children your own tranquilizers "just to keep them quiet."

Do not self-treat your insomnia with over-the-counter preparations, though they may seem to be harmless when taken occasionally. They usually contain one or more of the following: antihistamines, scopalamine, bromides, aspirin, vitamins. If taken over long periods without supervision, some such drugs, bromides, for example, may produce mental disorders. According to Drs. L.S. Goodman and A. Gilman, "From two to 10 per cent of the patients routinely admitted to psychiatric hospitals are found to be suffering from some degree of bromide intoxication."

SPECIFIC TIPS FOR OVERCOMING INSOMNIA

It is time now to give you specific tips to overcome your insomnia. I suggest that you read and reread these suggestions, for in some seemingly obscure and hidden phrase or sentence may be your own answer to the insomnia problem.

1. Remember that when you relax your muscles, you relax your nerves. Therefore try Dr. Jacobson's exercises for progressive relaxation of muscles. For example, try this one. Hold your arms by your sides with fists clenched for about a minute. Then let go gradually, taking another minute or two. Rest for several minutes, then repeat. Do this about three times. Relaxation gives a feeling not of actual numbness but of negativism. The opposite of tension. To become proficient you'll have to spend at least two to three hours daily practicing relaxation.
2. Never *try* to fall asleep.
3. Imagine that you are watching a pendulum and that your head is following it, swinging from side to side.
4. Try rolling your eyes in figures of eight until they get tired. Or try rolling them in complete circles a half-dozen times. Then reverse.
5. Breathe in slowly for ten seconds, hold air in for ten seconds, exhale for ten seconds. Repeat a few times.
6. Those who can't sleep in the dark carry over from

childhood a subconscious fear of the dark. Try sleeping by the light of a weak, blue bulb.

7. Try reversing your bed-position, putting your pillow where your feet were.

8. Try putting your mattress on the floor for a few nights.

9. Try counting each breath up to one hundred and then down to one.

10. Simply counting sheep is now considered an old-fashioned way to outwit insomnia. If you insist on counting them, then count every other one, the black sheep or every tenth sheep, which you should make jump backwards. Variations on sheep-counting are often successful.

11. Do not smoke before bedtime. The pipe that is supposed to soothe is often the culprit that keeps you awake.

12. Although an ounce of liquor or a glass of beer may give you a good night, more may keep you awake. Thus brandy sometimes makes the heart pound.

13. Let your imagination take over. For example, think of surf pounding on the beach.

14. Let your thoughts go back to the times when you were driving a long distance and became sleepy at the wheel. How difficult it was to keep your eyes open, and how well you slept when you pulled over to the side of the road.

15. Go to sleep by hi-fi or music on the radio.

16. It is important to try to go to bed at about the same time every night.

17. Try running through the alphabet, thinking of how many towns, flowers, etc., you can name, counting the oranges on each tree in an orange grove.

18. A good trick is to keep your eyes open against their desire to close. As the lids droop, force them open again until your eyes are so dry that it feels as if the Sandman had been

working overtime. You will rarely fall asleep if your eyes are well-lubricated. (The exception, of course, is when people cry themselves to sleep.)

19. I've heard that Jack Benny imagines he's painting a gigantic figure 3 on the side of a huge barn door to invite sleep. Any numeral up to ten might work as well for you. In many cases it's only a matter of self-hypnosis anyway.

20. Imagine that your hands and arms and legs are so heavy that you haven't the power and strength to lift them. If you can fool yourself into believing it, you will be asleep soon.

21. If you are an insomnophobe (a person afraid of not sleeping), all these suggestions will be of no avail unless you can face up to insomnia properly.

22. Do you use pajamas? Do you sleep in the raw? Experiment. Try a nightshirt or nightgown. Try sleeping with only uppers or lowers. (Speaking of uppers or lowers, this applies also to dentures. Some sleep better with them in; others with them out.)

23. Do you worry? You can't stop worrying, but you can learn to worry less. Resolve to do your worrying during the day. At night the problems assume diabolical proportions; during the day they look less ominous. If you really worry, you might try reading some humor before you go to bed. Robert Benchley has been known to cure at least one worrier of his problems, at least temporarily, and thereby to induce sleep.

24. If you suffer from a nasal allergy and sniff Benzedrine before bedtime and during the night, your insomnia may well be due to the waking powers of Benzedrine. If you stop using it, you may sleep—even though you will probably become a mouth-breather until the allergy wears off.

25. Since it takes the average person fifteen to thirty

minutes to fall asleep—though, of course, sometimes we are so in need for sleep that we're off within minutes—it is unfortunate that many people become restless if they do not fall asleep right away, for restlessness in itself produces insomnia. Be patient. Don't try to rush sleep. It will take its own good time about it.

26. Taking coffee before bedtime is a well-known, common cause of insomnia. Although for some people insomnia "may be in the mind," there is no question that the drink itself is responsible for much restlessness. Some people can sleep well after a half-dozen cups of coffee at night; others say that even the aroma of coffee before bedtime will keep them awake. "Caffeinism," due to either too much tea or too much coffee, causes rapid pulse, restlessness and insomnia. Caffeine stimulates nerve centers, increases mental activity, though most people say that taking tea before bedtime interferes less with their sleep than taking coffee. In any case, six cups of coffee a day are probably the maximum permissible for good health.

27. During menstruation and pregnancy sleep often becomes a problem that can be alleviated by the temporary use of sedatives.

28. In most stores you can buy sleep masks that help keep out the morning light and give you extra rest. Those overly sensitive to barking dogs, screeching brakes and other night noises can also buy ear-plugs. At specialty sleepshops there are scores of anti-insomnia contraptions such as chin straps, head and foot warmers, vibrators—but none is guaranteed to neutralize your sleeplessness.

29. One common cause of sleeplessness is lack of room in which to turn. Many married couples sleep in beds only a little over fifty inches in width. Is it any wonder they toss

fitfully when each sleeper really needs about forty inches of bed-width to himself?

30. Some people wake early in the morning simply because they are hungry. They are in the habit of having early dinners (around 5 P.M.) and do not eat anything until the following morning. Such persons should get into the habit of having a snack before bedtime.

31. Husbands and wives should try to develop similar sleep rhythms. One going to bed hours later than the other may upset the equilibrium of sleep as well as that of marriage.

32. A light massage before sleep is often helpful.

33. Try this exercise. Lie on your back and place your hands on your upper abdomen. Breathe slowly and deeply, keeping your eyes open wide. Hold your breath for a few seconds. Then, as you let it out slowly, close your eyes. Hold your breath again. Repeat until you feel drowsy. Or this one: raise your head from the pillow, breathe deeply (eight to ten breaths), then let your head drop heavily as you would a loaded basketball.

34. Puppies sleep with difficulty when their heads are lower than their bodies. Perhaps you will sleep better with an extra pillow.

35. If you have cold feet, wear socks.

36. If you feel a chill around your balding head, wear a nightcap. (Ignore the snickers of family or friends.)

37. Although the electric blanket is one of the great inventions of this century, keeping the temperature too high can cause insomnia.

38. Imitate sleep-breathing by breathing slowly and deeply—all the while, yoga-like, concentrating on your belly.

39. Try reading verses from the Bible.

40. Try fixing your attention on the tick of the clock.

41. Take a cold-air bath in the nude as Ben Franklin used to do. It was he who said: "Those who do not love trouble and can afford to have two beds, will find great luxury, in rising when awake in a hot bed, and going into a cool one."

42. Keep the bedroom temperature between sixty and sixty-five degrees.

43. Put a board under your mattress to prevent sagging. You do not have to complain of a bad back before you try this experiment.

44. Does rain-on-the-roof induce sleep? You can buy a Japanese gadget that imitates this sound.

TONGUE-IN-CHEEK METHOD

45. In my experience with patients the tongue-in-cheek method (which I will describe fully) has been most effective in overcoming stubborn insomnia. All that is necessary to master it is a modicum of perseverance.

For centuries man has been seeking many things assiduously: happiness, relief from pain, the answer to insomnia. For each there have been temporary, fleeting solutions. However, permanent ease has evaded us. Happiness is often illusory, pain returns and sleep remains a nightly enigma to millions.

Therefore, it is with full realization of the innocent treachery of sleep cures that I offer a method experience has shown me to be uniquely effective. Of all I have read about or tried personally (on myself and on patients) I know of none so effective.

I call it the "tongue-in-cheek" method of fighting insomnia because its basic formula is holding your tongue against your inner cheek. I invented it years ago, have tried it on hundreds and hundreds of patients and have proved its effectiveness.

I assume that you are an insomniac, twisting and turning and dreading the night, and that your thoughts, fed by some fearsome enzyme that stirs up your brain without letup, multiply and accelerate like thousands of restless amoebas bent only on reproduction.

As you lie there, I ask you to take inventory. Are your legs tense? Your arms? Your neck? Perhaps, but not invariably. How are your jaws? Your eyes? Your tongue?

Undoubtedly you have heard these admonitions: unclamp your jaws; separate your teeth; try to relax your eyes. But have you ever been asked about the position of your tongue?

It is unlikely that you have, until this moment. Yet there is the key that may unlock your bedroom door to a good night's sleep. As you lie fully awake ask yourself, "Where is the tip of my tongue?"

If you are an insomniac, I will tell you where it is: pressing hard against the roof of your mouth or against the back ridge of your upper teeth.

Your immediate task is to find ways and means to relax the tense muscles around your jaw. Not until your tongue tires and drops back, relaxed, and your teeth have unlocked, will you find sleep.

There is one way to accomplish this effectively: the tongue-in-cheek method. Try it tonight. In many persons it works immediately. In stubborn insomniacs it brings sleep only after a few nights or weeks of practice. It is simple, but its effectiveness will depend upon your conscientious application of its principles.

Step 1. (General Considerations)

Review basic essentials. Ask yourself the following questions and take the appropriate measures to remedy situations:

Is my bed as comfortable as possible? Does it have good springs? A comfortable mattress? Pillows that are neither too soft nor too hard? Appropriate covers (not too light in cold months and not too heavy in summer)? Is the room temperature correct? Is the air circulation effective and free from direct drafts? Are the bedclothes loosened at the foot of the bed to allow easy, free, nonrestrictive foot movement? Have I taken coffee or tea directly before bedtime? Have I smoked? Have I overloaded my stomach? Am I really comfortable in a double bed or do I need a single bed?

General considerations such as these are essential before you can expect specific remedial action from any procedure.

Step 2. (Eye Relaxation and Rhythmic Breathing)

Often the insomniac is awake for hours before he realizes he has been lying with his eyes forcibly closed. It is natural to keep your eyes closed when you are trying hard to fall asleep, but keeping them closed has the opposite effect: it guarantees wakefulness.

Overcome eye tenseness by forcibly keeping your eyes open, staring into the darkness. The resulting dryness of the eyeballs is an invitation to sleepiness. Periods of eye-closure following enforced staring will become longer and longer. Just before you feel you may be dropping off to sleep, regulate your breathing so that you breathe in deeply when your eyes are open and breathe out when they are closed. This rhythmic cooperation between eyes and lungs will at last propel you into the sleepy state. It is impossible to fall asleep while you are unconsciously tensing your eyelids. The open-closed sequence, combined with studied breathing, will prevent tenseness.

Step 3. (Tongue-in-Cheek Method)

You will need to experiment. As you lie still wakeful, ask yourself, "Where is the tip of my tongue?" As I said earlier, it is likely pressing hard against the roof of your mouth or along the back ridge of your upper teeth. Until you break this "contact," you will be unable to relax completely, and Step 2, although helpful, may not work properly.

Therefore, disengage your tongue from these two points of pressure-contact. Immediately you will find that tenseness begins to disappear. Unfortunately, you will find that within seconds your tongue-tip will have found its previous pressure point, and wakefulness will have returned.

The solution to this problem revolves around whether you can keep the tip of your tongue away from the roof of your mouth or the back of your upper teeth. Doing it is simple.

Gently slide your tongue-tip between your teeth against your inner cheek. Relaxation will come immediately. Put the tip of your little finger between your teeth. You will find that your tongue has comfortably separated the uppers from the lowers. No longer are they clenched in tension. Your lower jaw has dropped at least a half-inch. This in itself produces relaxation.

If you find that you fall asleep within minutes, it is not necessary to refine this method of sleep production. In any case, individual experience will prescribe the method of choice: if you lie on your right side, place your tongue-tip in your left cheek; if on your left side, place it in your right cheek; if on your back or abdomen, slide the tip of your tongue over the front of your lower teeth into the smooth groove between lower lip and lower teeth. There are no definite "left side," "right side" rules. As you fall off to sleep, your tongue will assume its normal position.

This tongue-in-cheek maneuver has helped hundreds of insomniacs who had unsuccessfully fought the battle for years. They returned to me astounded and relieved that such a simple method could overcome so stubborn an opponent. Combined with eye-stare and rhythmic breathing and the eye-open, eye-closed exercise, I have found the tongue-maneuver to be the most effective method I know.

I offer no scientific reason for its workability. All I can say is that disengaging the tongue-tip from the roof of the mouth seems to remove some sort of contact—thus promoting relaxation rather than tenseness. But whether the contact is electrical, psychological or anatomical in nature, I will not even venture to guess.

But I can promise that my tongue-in-cheek antidote is often quite effective against the poison of insomnia. If all other methods have failed, it deserves a decent trial period.

Sleep well.

20 | Closing Note: The Outlook

MY FRIEND, Mr. V., said, "Wouldn't it be wonderful if we didn't have to sleep at all? Think of all the time we would save."

People who are thankful they can have at least seven or eight hours of forgetfulness in sleep, oblivious of their many trials and troubles, would disagree. They say that sixteen hours of wakefulness each day is about all they want or need.

If we say we are actually alive only when we are aware of what goes on about us, that is, we are awake, it is true that we "waste" one-third of our lives in sleep. Instead of living to the biblical three-score-and-ten, we live only two-thirds of seventy years (the other third being forever lost in sleep). So, I asked myself, will we ever be able to "live" that lost third.

The answer, of course, is yes. One day, when we know exactly what sleep is, scientists will invent a sleep-saving machine. At the end of a full day you will connect the machine to some part of your anatomy and press a button. You will immediately fall into a deep sleep for ten to fifteen minutes. At the end of the period, you will be awakened as refreshed as if you had just had eight hours of natural sleep.

Fantastic? Ridiculous? No. Such a development is far from impossible in this marvelous age of electronics. Not too many years from now our grandchildren may wonder why we even doubted such a thing could come to pass.

Meanwhile, however, until such a wondrous, electronic

apparatus takes over to produce concentrated, artificial sleep, I suggest that you follow the Sleepmanship techniques I have outlined in this book. Take advantage of everything you know in the present. Tomorrow is too late to overcome tonight's insomnia.

Index

Adolescents, sleep needs of, 34, 36
Adults, sleep needs of, 34, 160, 185
Allergies, 4, 131-36, 199
Alvarez, Walter C., 62
Anemia, 2, 55
Angina pectoris, 104, 165
Anxiety, 2, 4, 20, 74, 75, 91-94, 95, 97, 105-118, 140-42, 161, 163, 188
Arteriosclerosis, 96, 99, 160
Asthma, 131, 134
Atherosclerosis, 96, 99, 137
Azima, H., 144

Bailey, M.A., 66
Basal metabolism, 21, 43, 130
Baude, 35
Beds and bedding, 4, 80-84, 135, 152, 157, 171, 176, 190, 200-201, 204
Berg, Charles, 61
Blackwell, Elizabeth, 77
Blood pressure, 20-21, 24-25, 66, 160, 165
Braines, 38
Brande, Dorothea, 113
Breuer, Joseph, 155

Callahan, Robert, 60
Carrel, Alexis, 185
Cataplexy, 42-43
Children, sleep needs of, 34-36, 42, 45, 160
Coughlin, Robert, 75
Critchley, Macdonald, 45, 49

Damrau, Adeline M., 159
Damrau, Frederic, 159
Darwin, 169
Dermatitis, 136
Devlin, Joseph, 165
Diabetes, 118
Digestion, 21
Dorfman, Wilfred, 143
Dreams, 4, 21, 22, 25, 43, 57-64, 104, 152, 153, 161; *see also* Nightmares

Ekbom, K.A., 49, 54, 56
Elderly, sleep needs of, 36-38, 154, 155
Electroencephalogram, 22, 23-24
Emmons, William H., 168
English, O. Spurgeon, 61

Fatigue, 1, 2, 9-10, 14, 15, 16, 43, 46, 73, 99, 117-18, 127-28, 156, 158, 160, 161, 162, 169
Fisher, Charles, 169
Foote, E.B., 17, 78
Freud, 58-59, 62, 155

Gelineau, 42
Giles, Ray, 159
Gilman, A., 197
Goodman, L.S., 197

Hamburg, W. Robert, 63
Hamilton, Lyle H., 60
Hay fever, 132-36
Heart acceleration, 91-92
Heart ailments, 4, 91-104, 118, 165
Heart skips, 94, 128, 140
Hernia, 4, 163-64
Hertzler, Arthur E., 143
Hypertension, 98-102
Hyperthyroidism, 4, 128-30; *see also* Thyroid disorders
Hypothyroidism, 40, 43, 44, 118, 127-28; *see also* Thyroid disorders

Jacobson, Edmund, 184, 197
Jordan, R.L., 69

Kahn, B.I., 69
Kasinoff, B.H., 66
Kelly, Frances P., 60
Kingman, R., 162
Kitay, William, 193
Kleitman, Nathaniel, 15, 25, 59, 62, 157

Laird, D.A., 37
Leg cramps, 163
Leg jitters, 48-56, *see also* Restless Leg syndrome
Leibniz, G.W., 59
Liddy, Emma, 159

McDougall, William, 193-94
Mann, George, 60
Menopause, 4, 137-38
Mental disorders, 4, 20, 38, 63, 67, 102, 128, 139-48, 154-55, 161, 165
Miller, M.M., 163
Murray, John M., 61
Muscle tone, 21, 23, 43
Myxedema, 128

Naps, 4, 26-27, 36-37, 38, 42, 100-101, 153, 156, 157, 159, 162, 192-94
Narcolepsy, 4, 39-47, 166
Neuroses, 13, 42, 44-45, 46, 69, 74, 189
Nightmares, 4, 21, 63, 64-68, 69, 104, 178

Orgasmolepsy, 42
Orthopnea (difficulty in breathing), 100

Parkinson's disease, 4, 164
Prostate disease, 4, 36, 164
Pulse rate, 21, 23, 63, 160

Rapid eye movement (REM) 25, 59, 63, 104
Reflexes, 21
Relaxing, 184, 186-87, 192-206
Respiration, 21, 23, 24, 25, 63, 201
Restless Leg syndrome, 4, 48-56, 177
Rheumatic fever, 102-103, 132

Sadger, J. Isador, 68
St. John, John and Diana, 167
Scarlett, E.P., 86-87
Schwab, Robert S., 117

Seashore, Carl E., 159
Selye, Hans, 168
Simon, Charles W., 168
Sleep center, brain's, 9, 15
Sleeping pills, 4, 22, 56, 95, 101, 103, 124, 136, 140, 146-48, 152, 160, 171, 178, 194-97
Sleep learning, 168
Sleep rhythms, 25-27, 30, 32-38, 155, 201
Sleep stages, 21, 22-25, 59, 61, 63
Sleep therapy, 143-45
Sleepwalking, 4, 68-69
Snoring, 4, 70-71, 80, 153, 176, 190

Teeth grinding (bruxism), 66, 68, 177
Temperature, body, 21, 23, 33-34, 63
Theories of sleep, 3, 4, 5, 9, 13-15, 17-18, 29, 38
Thyroid disorders, 125-30; *see also* Hypothyroidism; Hyperthyroidism
Tiller, Philip M., Jr., 37
Tranquilizers, 4, 56, 100, 112, 124, 136, 137, 138, 140, 152, 155, 165, 195-96
Tridon, Andre, 59
Tuberculosis, 118
Turning in sleep, 21, 22, 24, 25, 169

Ulcers, 4, 119-24, 142

Wagner, C.P., 43
Waking center, brain's, 15
Weiss, Edward, 66
Weiss, H.R., 66
Whitehead, S.B., 25
Willis, Thomas, 50